JF

Recent Titles in the

CONTEMPORARY WORLD ISSUES
Series

Domestic Violence and Abuse: A Reference Handbook
Laura L. Finley

Torture and Enhanced Interrogation: A Reference Handbook
Christina Ann-Marie DiEdoardo

Racism in America: A Reference Handbook
Steven L. Foy

Waste Management: A Reference Handbook
David E. Newton

Sexual Harassment: A Reference Handbook
Merril D. Smith

The Climate Change Debate: A Reference Handbook
David E. Newton

Voting Rights in America: A Reference Handbook
Richard A. Glenn and Kyle L. Kreider

Modern Slavery: A Reference Handbook
Christina G. Villegas

Race and Sports: A Reference Handbook
Rachel Laws Myers

World Oceans: A Reference Handbook
David E. Newton

First Amendment Freedoms: A Reference Handbook
Michael C. LeMay

Medicare and Medicaid: A Reference Handbook
Greg M. Shaw

Organic Food and Farming: A Reference Handbook
Shauna M. McIntyre

Civil Rights and Civil Liberties in America: A Reference Handbook
Michael C. LeMay

GMO Food: A Reference Handbook, Second Edition
David E. Newton

Books in the **Contemporary World Issues** series address vital issues in today's society such as genetic engineering, pollution, and biodiversity. Written by professional writers, scholars, and nonacademic experts, these books are authoritative, clearly written, up-to-date, and objective. They provide a good starting point for research by high school and college students, scholars, and general readers as well as by legislators, businesspeople, activists, and others.

Each book, carefully organized and easy to use, contains an overview of the subject, a detailed chronology, biographical sketches, facts and data and/or documents and other primary source material, a forum of authoritative perspective essays, annotated lists of print and nonprint resources, and an index.

Readers of books in the Contemporary World Issues series will find the information they need in order to have a better understanding of the social, political, environmental, and economic issues facing the world today.

Pregnancy and Birth

A REFERENCE HANDBOOK

Keisha L. Goode and Barbara Katz Rothman

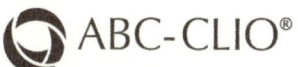

ABC-CLIO®

An Imprint of ABC-CLIO, LLC
Santa Barbara, California • Denver, Colorado

Library of Congress Cataloging-in-Publication Data

Names: Goode, Keisha L., author. | Rothman, Barbara Katz, author.
Title: Pregnancy and birth : a reference handbook / Keisha L. Goode and Barbara Katz Rothman.
Other titles: Contemporary world issues.
Description: Santa Barbara, California : ABC-CLIO, [2021] | Series: Contemporary world issues | Includes bibliographical references and index.
Identifiers: LCCN 2020047762 (print) | LCCN 2020047763 (ebook) | ISBN 9781440869211 (hardcover ; alk. paper) | ISBN 9781440869228 (ebook)
Subjects: MESH: Pregnancy | Parturition | Maternal Welfare | United States
Classification: LCC RG525 (print) | LCC RG525 (ebook) | NLM WQ 200 AA1 | DDC 618.2—dc23
LC record available at https://lccn.loc.gov/2020047762
LC ebook record available at https://lccn.loc.gov/2020047763

ISBN: 978-1-4408-6921-1 (print)
      978-1-4408-6922-8 (ebook)

25 24 23 22 21   1 2 3 4 5

This book is also available as an eBook.

ABC-CLIO
An Imprint of ABC-CLIO, LLC

ABC-CLIO, LLC
147 Castilian Drive
Santa Barbara, California 93117
www.abc-clio.com

This book is printed on acid-free paper ∞

Manufactured in the United States of America

Americans talk as if pregnancy is a medical condition to be diagnosed and managed and of babies as "coming into the world," arriving as if from some other place, packages "delivered" and brought home from the hospital. The United States' dominant medical model of pregnancy and birth values systematization, management, efficiency, and control. This does not reflect the normal physiologic process of birth nor the interdependent nature of human existence. Where is the person in the body? Where is the person in the technocratic cascade of medical interventions? What emotional and physical connections between birthing person and baby are disrupted?

This wide-ranging book introduces readers to U.S. pregnancy and birth from a person-centered, Reproductive Justice perspective. All pregnancies end, whether by live birth with one's gestational parent, surrogacy, or adoption. They may also end by miscarriage, abortion, or stillbirth. This book introduces readers to these experiences and outcomes using historical account, empirical data, and personal essays. We maintain that how a society primarily treats pregnant and birthing people is a demonstration of how it values human life.

The womb is the baby's first environment. The baby's transition from the womb to the world—the birthing process, setting, and people present—is our first demonstration of care, love, and value for baby, birthing person, and family. How we are born, and what we are born into, matters. Birth, the subsequent growth and development of children, and the raising of a younger generation, with all of the familial, communal, and social resources required, are universal aspects of human existence. It is important for our readers to understand that our use of the terms "pregnant person" and "birthing person" throughout the book is intentional. Not all people that have wombs, get pregnant, or give birth, identify as women. Thus, wherever possible, we use birthing person, a gender-inclusive term, to refer to cisgender, transgender, gender non-conforming, genderqueer, and non-binary people.

This book provides readers with a starting point in understanding aspects of the beauty and complexities of pregnancy and birth in the United States. The following summaries of chapter content provide guidance on where to find particular information:

- Chapter 1, "Background and History," offers a broad overview of the development of pregnancy and birth in the United States. This chapter is organized into two parts. The first part demonstrates how pregnancy has come to be understood in American culture, and the second part focuses on the history of birthing practices with specific attention to the status of midwifery and its relationship to both law and obstetric dominance.
- Chapter 2, "Problems, Controversies, and Solutions," discusses seven key issues that, whether in mass media or academic or mainstream literature, have not gained the urgent attention they deserve. The birthing outcomes and experiences of Indigenous peoples and transgender people, in particular, have been largely overlooked. This chapter addresses these issues along, with the professionalization of caring, highlighting media representations of pregnancy and birth, the high costs associated with the perinatal health care system, and the importance of the U.S. census toward allocating more resources. The chapter concludes with centering Reproductive Justice, as a framework and as a practice, as the primary solution to addressing the problems and controversies discussed in the chapter, and throughout this book.

- Chapter 3, "Perspectives," comprises 10 essays written by parents, providers, scholars, policy experts, and activists, who offer their perspectives on specific components of pregnancy and birth in the United States not otherwise featured in other chapters of this book.
- Chapter 4, "Profiles," highlights some of the many influential individuals and organizations that have changed the direction of, or contributed to, the understanding and experiences of pregnancy and birth in the United States.
- Chapter 5, "Data and Documents," presents a range of data and research findings on U.S. birth statistics, with some aggregation by race/ethnicity and provider. The documents section compiles excerpts of relevant historical documents and other primary texts created by professional associations, activists, lawmakers, government agencies, and scholars that situate the topic within a broader social, political, and cultural context.
- Chapter 6, "Resources," offers an annotated list of books, articles, and other sources for further research into the medicalization of pregnancy and birth; assisted reproductive technology and surrogacy; media representations of pregnancy and birth; racial and ethnic birth disparities and inequities; and, experiences of pregnant and birthing LGBTQ people and families.
- Chapter 7, "Chronology," presents an annotated, chronological list of some dates and events that have been pivotal to the history of pregnancy and birth in the United States.

This book concludes with a succinct glossary of relevant terms for reader reference.

Acknowledgments

We wish to thank Allie McDonough for her stellar work as a research assistant. She has meticulously supported this work, all driven by her commitment to introducing students to a perspective on U.S. pregnancy and birth that is person-centered. We wish to also thank Marisa Mendez Marthallar, for her work on supporting the research and organization of this book's resources, data, and documents. We are so grateful to Rhonda Grantham for her contributions to chapter 2; to our essay contributors featured in chapter 3; and to Linda Janet Holmes, Jennie Joseph, Mary Lawlor, Patricia Loftman, Shafia Monroe, Suzy Myers, and Haguerenesh Tesfa and Jamarah Amani of the National Black Midwives Alliance for their contributions to the profiles featured in chapter 4. Thank you to Ken Ingram for his patience and tireless copy editing. Finally, our eternal gratitude goes to all birth and Reproductive Justice workers, activists, educators, researchers, and organizations; thank you for all that you do.

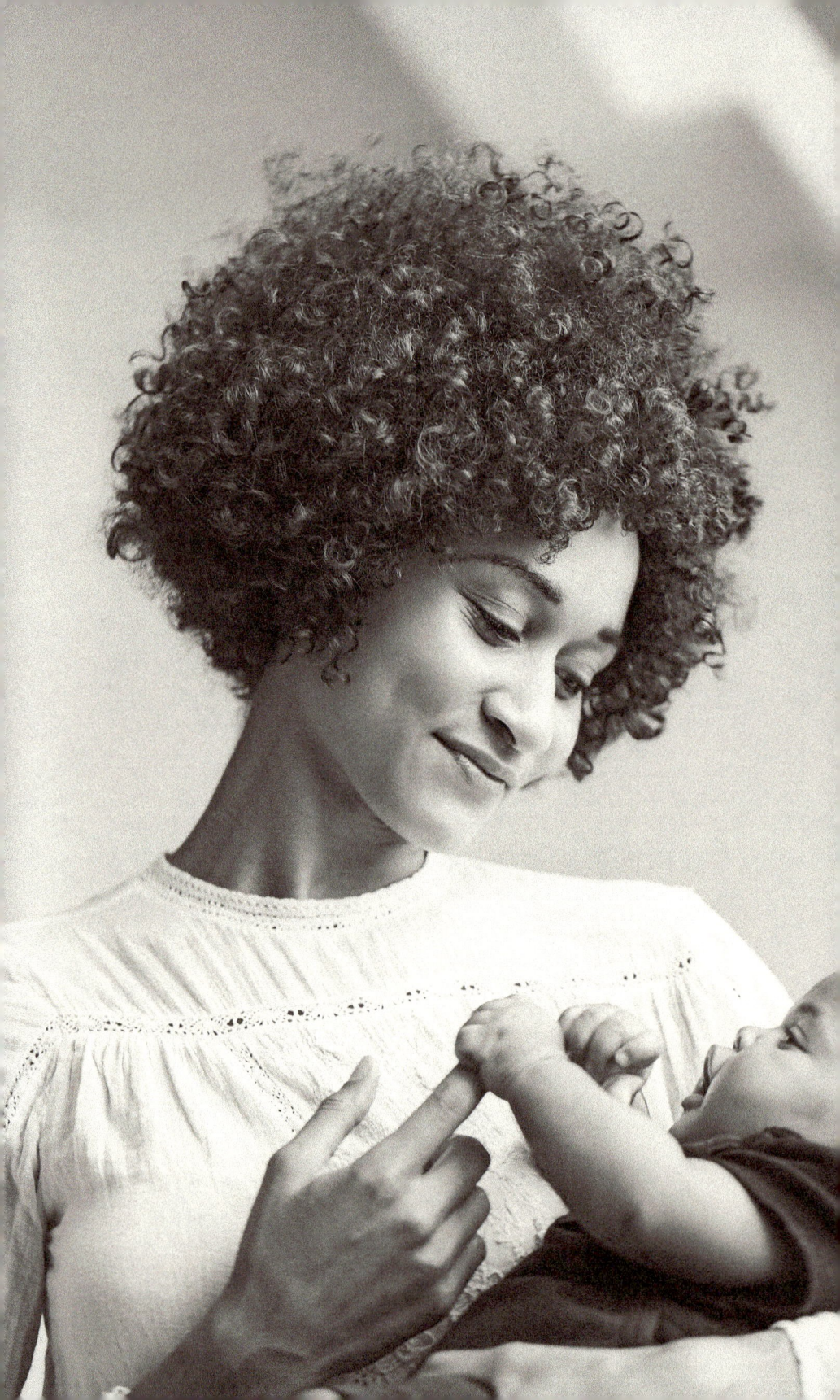

Introduction

The history of pregnancy and birth is of course complex, drawing on many different factors and comprising many different histories. Here we focus on two particular aspects. In part I, we show how pregnancy has come to be understood in American culture and how that has changed over time with social and scientific changes, culminating in a focus and fascination with the fetus. In part II, we focus on the history of birthing practices with a focus on the status of midwifery and its relationship to both law and obstetric dominance.

Part I: The Development of the Fetal Patient

The concept and very meaning of pregnancy is deeply rooted in cultural and social structures. Anthropologists distinguish matrilineal from patrilineal societies, those that believe that people are the descendants of women and those that believe people come from men. This, it is important to note, is different than the idea of patriarchal or matriarchal societies, those ruled by men or by women, respectively. If a society is matrilineal but patriarchal, men still rule, but it would be the maternal uncle and not the father of a young man, for example, who will

---

Newborn bonding. (Monkey Business Images/Dreamstime.com)

have control over the kinds of work his nephew may do and who will decide whom his niece may marry.

American society grew out of the Judeo-Christian heritage, in which God is the "father," and people are the descendants and products of men. The Bible claims that it is the "seed of Abraham" to whom God made his promises. In this perspective, children grow out of the seeds of men, which are planted in the bodies of women. From this comes the old-fashioned idea of women as vessels or containers. In a matrilineal perspective, people trace their heritage back through the bodies of women; future generations are in women, not planted there by men. Naming practices generally follow those rules. In American society, even today, children are generally given the last names of their fathers, and up until very recently, it was understood that, for example, "Mrs. John Smith bore John Smith Jr."

The early development of science followed from this patriarchal, hetero-normative perspective. One of the first uses of the microscope was to examine sperm, and Nicolaas Hartsoeker, a Dutch scientist, drew what he thought he saw in the head of a sperm in 1694: a little person. He used the term *homunculus*, Latin for "little man," to describe what he perceived. In contrast, the first description of the human ovum was by a German scientist in 1827. Through the 1700s and on into the 1800s, there were *ovists* and *spermists*, those who thought the future baby was in the ovum and those who thought it was in the sperm, respectively. In 1875, Oscar Hertwig showed a sperm head fusing with female genetic material in sea urchins, and the idea of two genetic parents contributing equally entered our thinking. One hundred three years later, the first baby was born as a result of in vitro fertilization (IVF), a baby created by doing the fusing, or *fertilization*, outside of the human body.

Contemporary science has now pointed out that the maternal genetic contribution also includes the mitochondrial DNA, a genetic contribution that does not come from the nucleus of the ovum but its surrounding body. When a person cannot produce a healthy egg cell, the nucleus of their egg can replace that in another person's ovum, and a baby can be begun through IVF. Interestingly, has been called a "three-parent" baby—counting three genetic contributors and not even including the pregnancy as a part of the creation of the baby.

American practice and beliefs about pregnancy continue to reflect both patrilineal and patriarchal beliefs. Once the seeds of women were recognized as equal to that of men, children became "half his and half hers," and the place they were "planted" has little significance. Pregnancy, seen through this perspective, hardly exists: babies are said to "arrive" and "enter the world" and to be "delivered." Pregnancy is called "expecting a baby" rather than growing one. Of course, birthing people do not feel babies "arrive" or "be delivered" when they push them out of their bodies.

That dismissal of pregnancy as a present state, rather than a state of expectation, began to shift as the fetus was made visible through new technologies. Early use of x-rays showed fetal skeletons, and x-rays were used from the 1920s for confirmation of pregnancy as well as diagnostic imaging for placental placement, fetal position, twins, fetal size, etc. There was increasing concern about the dangers of radiation for fetal development. By the mid-1970s, evidence demonstrated that radiation contributed to miscarriage, leukemia, and other cancers. Other imaging technologies were being developed, and the major breakthrough was ultrasound, which entered obstetric practice in the late 1970s and quickly became routine. Ultrasound imaging provides a more photographic image than x-rays. One can see the fetal features, the face becomes recognizable, and the images can be seen in real time; the fetus can be watched as it moves and breathes within the pregnant person's body.

This was not the first imaging of fetuses that enabled the public to see them as "unborn babies." In 1965, Swedish photographer Lennart Nilsson published photographs of fetuses in

LIFE magazine. The article was called "Drama of Life before Birth," but the fetuses whose images were shown were in fact not "before birth" but after miscarriage or abortion. They looked like sleeping babies, but they were in fact deceased fetuses. The images stayed with people, and the idea of the fetus as baby, the fetus present but invisible, became part of American culture. And it became very much part of dominant American medical culture.

Electronic fetal monitoring was introduced in the 1960s and 1970s to continuously monitor fetal heart tones; rather than having a midwife, nurse, or physician come to the side of the laboring people and listen through their abdomen, the person could be strapped to a machine, and the fetal heart rate could be read at a central location. The monitoring was first introduced for high-risk pregnancies, but as is often the case, the new technology quickly became standard management. An electrode could be screwed into the fetal scalp, and fetal blood could also be continuously monitored from a nurses' station or other location away from the labor room. Research evidence does not indicate that this brings an improvement in outcome over direct intermittent auscultation, the listening to the fetus that earlier caregivers were able to do. It also increased the idea that the separately monitored and managed fetus was a separate patient from the birthing person.

Separate specialties of fetal surgery were being developed, though their success rates have been quite low. More significant than the development of the separate specialty of fetal management was that the field of obstetrics began to define the fetus as its prime and most vulnerable patient. The law began to work with medicine to enforce control over pregnant people's bodies and lives in the presumed interest of the fetus. People have been arrested and tried for behavior that a physician claimed caused miscarriage. People have been subjected to forced, court-ordered cesarean sections. In some cases, "nature intervened," and people had successful vaginal births before the scheduled cesareans. Some of these cases were brought to higher courts, though even if the person "won," it was far too late to stop the forced surgery.

The routine use of ultrasound to learn more and more about the fetus in utero, including its presumed sex through examining the shape of its observable genitalia, has brought us the fetus as a named, sexed being. Fetal images are now quite common, but those images erase the birthing person's body entirely. In fact, almost all of those images have been turned upside down to show the fetus upright, as a baby would be held—unless it was in the relatively rare breech position—which would mean the birthing person was standing on their head. The fetus has been made more visible and more real. Person-centered care is required to resist the dominant recreation of birthing people as fetal containers.

Part II: Birthing Practices

Birthing practices have continuously evolved throughout American history, beginning with the arrival of the colonizers who stole land and cultural practices from Indigenous peoples (see more in chapter 2), and into the present day. Throughout the early period in America, birthing was oriented toward family and community, primarily dominated and defined by women, and occurred within the physical and emotional space of the home. It was based on women's knowledge and experience that had been passed down through generations of midwives, women in the community who were the recognized experts in birth. After a birth, midwives and the other women in the family and community cared for both the baby and the birthing person, and it was not until days or weeks later that friends and family would visit and sometimes have a christening or naming ritual for the baby. Pregnant people knew labor signs and when to call for a midwife, neighbors, friends, and family, who would bring things to help ease the labor, such as tea, herbal preparations, syrup, or other natural remedies. The job of the midwife was to take charge and help the birthing person get as comfortable as possible (Mather 1972; Leighton 1986).

The history of Black midwifery in the United States extends to the knowledge, skills and culture that midwives of African descent had prior to forceful capture in enslavement on American shores in the seventeenth century. In the cultural imagination, U.S. Black midwifery begins in the South with the "granny" midwives. There is often a historical assumption that grand midwives relied solely on "divine intervention" because of "the call" to be a midwife (Haynes 2003; Lee 1996). Although the calling and a connection to the spiritual realm may be central to some cultural midwifery, it does not follow that grand midwives practiced without knowledge of and skill in pregnancy and birth. "To be accepted in the slave quarter, a woman had to gain the confidence of other slaves by demonstrating an aptitude or calling. A woman who did not have the support of her people would not have attempted to assist in childbirth" (Schwartz 2006). These midwives attended to other enslaved people and plantation mistresses in birth, reproductive care, and healing well into the postemancipation mid-twentieth century (Luke 2018; Lee 1996; Mongeau, Smith, and Maney 1961; Tunc 2010). Granny midwives literally aided in the building of community by caring for and supporting people throughout pregnancy and during birth as they brought forth new life. Midwives also reportedly acted as what Patricia Hill Collins (2000) called "othermothers," which was common in communities of color, specifically the Black community; they were biologically and socially related women that provided care, nurturance, and empowerment to children, other women, and families. The term *granny*, however, is contested, as it echoes connotations of passivity and servility and is closely related to the image of the mammy, a caretaker for slave owners and their children. Neither the term *granny* nor *mammy* portrays the experience and skills these women had. The cultural beliefs about women in general, and Black women in particular, is that they act on "instinct" rather than learning, which dismisses all the experience and tacit knowledge they shared and taught generation to generation. We will use the term *grand midwives* in the remainder of this chapter.

Enslavers and the newly developing physicians collaborated in efforts to increase fertility among enslaved people, beginning in puberty and continuing throughout their reproductive years. Burgeoning obstetricians and gynecologists brutally and inhumanely experimented on enslaved women (Cooper-Owens 2017; Kapsalis 1997). Doing so allowed them to participate in active medical debates about perinatal and women's health, that were beginning in Europe and the northern United States (Briggs 2000; Edwards-Ingram 2001; Kobrin 1966; Schwartz 2006).

In the early seventeenth century, in England, the barber-surgeon Peter Chamberlen developed the obstetrical forceps, an instrument that enabled its user to deliver a child mechanically. The Chamberlen family kept the forceps secret for three generations for their own financial gain and only let it be known that they possessed some way of preventing piecemeal extraction of an impacted fetus. The right to use instruments still resided exclusively with men, and when the Chamberlen finally sold their design it was for the use of barber-surgeons and not generally available to midwives.

It has frequently been assumed that the forceps were an enormous breakthrough in improving perinatal care, but this has hardly been demonstrated, and, in retrospect, it seems unlikely. Physicians and surgeons did not have the opportunity to observe and learn the rudiments of normal physiologic birth because men were unwelcome at births. They were therefore at a decided disadvantage in handling difficult births. Unlike in the days prior to the invention of forceps, when a barber-surgeon was called in only if all hope of a live birth was abandoned, midwives in the seventeenth and eighteenth centuries were increasingly encouraged and instructed to call in the barber-surgeon prophylactically whenever a birth became difficult. This is part and parcel of the larger pattern of the history of midwifery: midwives lost autonomy and control of their work to physicians, and obstetric dominance allocated birthing people according to notions of appropriate "territory." Physicians carved out pathological and abnormal births as their territory. They eventually went on to define pregnancy, contraception, abortion, infertility, and birth itself as inherently pathological and abnormal. This contributed to the attempted disenfranchisement of midwives, but midwives have still persisted.

The first cesarean section recorded in which both birthing person and baby survived was performed by an Irish midwife, Mary Dunally (Donnison 1977, 49). Wherever one encounters this story, Dunally is inevitably described as "illiterate," and the home had a dirt floor. Of course, there was no training manual she could have read nor a book of instructions. There were no antiseptic hospitals with sterilized floors. She understood the body, understood the position of the baby, and presumably knew how to sew. As the development of basic anatomical knowledge and increased understanding of the processes of reproduction grew, surgeons of the 1700s eventually began to develop formal training programs in childbirth management. Women, including midwives, were systematically excluded from such programs. Women were not trained because women were believed to be inherently incompetent. The result was a widening disparity between midwives and surgeons. As new and sophisticated techniques were developed by the men, they were kept from the women (Donnison 1977).

Once the surgeon or physician is deemed necessary "in case something goes wrong," the midwife becomes dependent on the physician and their goodwill for "backup" services. If a midwife decides a person needs medical assistance—a cesarean section or a drug only physicians have the right to prescribe—they need the physician to accept their transfer or call for request. When physicians want to compete with midwives for clients, all they have to do is withhold these backup services by refusing to come to the aid of a midwife who calls for medical assistance.

This is a pattern that began in the earliest days of the barber-surgeon and continues today.

Continuing through the early 1800s, physicians began to use ergot, a fungus that can be a potent oxytocic; it was used to speed up and intensify contractions. Dr. John Stearns learned about this from a midwife; however, he did not learn how to properly prepare it, and, as a result, he both helped and harmed birthing people and fetuses throughout the nineteenth century. During this time, opium was also used for pain relief, which often halted contractions, and by mid-century, chloroform was used as an anesthetic to erase pain and painful memories (Bogdan 1978). Since the seventeenth century, midwifery has truly been under attack in Europe, beginning with the barber-surgeons, who held a monopoly on the use of forceps when they were first invented. Other male physicians entered the field, claiming that women lacked the necessary competence. In a male-dominated society, men had only to assert their competence to have it recognized. But the burgeoning field of obstetrics cost the lives of birthing people and babies, who could have been saved at the hands of a midwife.

In the eighteenth- and nineteenth-century United States, enslaved birthing people were further dehumanized as breeders by enslavers, and frequent pregnancies were encouraged to maximize labor and eventual profits. Births then occurred in their quarters, with friends, family, and a midwife. At this time, midwives were the most skilled people on the plantation, and those skills were acknowledged by their owners: enslaved midwives were called upon for the births by slave owners' wives (Norton 1996; White 1987). Nonetheless, obstetric dominance of birth was beginning to take a strong hold. In the beginning of the nineteenth century, the majority (approximately 70–90 percent) of white plantation births were attended by midwives (enslaved or white); by 1860, an estimated 40–50 percent of plantation mistresses were delivered by physicians. At first, physicians were called as a last resort, just in case a birth became difficult, but in the nineteenth century, physicians increasingly began to handle all births—replacing midwives as the chief attendant. They were called in because they were male, they were credentialed, and they could do "something" when women and midwives, it was believed, could not; childbirth was suddenly seen to need medical attention and intervention. This pattern of increase continued well into the twentieth century (Tunc 2010, 411–412). For Black women, however, the majority of births continued to be attended by midwives. Dramatic intervention tactics from physicians were commonly used during the late eighteenth and early nineteenth centuries and included the forceps (which were used to save the lives of both infant and the mother under hopeless conditions), venesection or bloodletting (used to restart contractions), and tobacco enemas if the bloodletting did not work (Bogdan 1978).

Post-emancipation, these formerly enslaved midwives, along with other midwives of color and European immigrant midwives, primarily remained in the South. In a culture of dehumanization and oppression, midwives (also dehumanized and oppressed themselves) operating as birth workers, healers, and othermothers, served an important role as skilled caretakers and nurturers. The latter half of the nineteenth century, however, brought a fundamental "scientific" shift to traditional midwifery practice. Beginning in the 1830s, though becoming popularized in the 1860s and 1870s, white physicians and public health reformers developed a "sanitary science" that "linked organic chemical impurities or ferment's in the air and water to the rising incidence of diseases such as cholera and typhoid fever" (Tomes 1997, 37). An increasing number of scientists extended the premise of sanitary science to conclude that the roots of varying human disease were in fact living microorganisms, or germs, thereby cementing the "germ theory of disease." The germ theory became widely proselytized by the medical and public health establishment. This sparked a widespread obsession with the cleanliness of American homes to prevent deadly diseases. It was the responsibility of mothers, and women more generally, to ensure the safety, sanitation, and cleanliness of the nation by mothering scientifically (Feldstein 2000; Wilkie 2003). Physicians and hospitals became definitive symbols of safety, sanitation, and cleanliness—even though hospitals and physician offices were the most dangerous sites for the spread of infection. The conventional thought regarding the ignorance, incompetence, unsafety, and uncleanliness of midwives of the time cannot be disassociated from racism, and specifically anti-Blackness.

The discourse of sanitary science and the germ theory of disease positioned midwives—distanced from the credentialed legitimacy of physicians and the perceived precision of modern scientific knowledge and application—in a very vulnerable position. The American Medical Association (AMA) was founded in 1847. By the end of the nineteenth century and into the early twentieth century, the allopathic physicians it represented, and not the "competing sections of healers" vying for "public recognition and support and for the financial rewards of medical practice," were institutionally represented and politically successful (Brickman 1983, 67).

Health and fertility have always been constrained by social forces of colonization and racism. For more than a century after the Civil War, the work of midwives was under attack by reformers because, in addition to childbirth, they also performed abortions and provided other forms of health care. Thus, the necessity of secrecy surrounding health care for Black women continued long after slavery had ended. J. Marion Sims, proclaimed to be the "father" of modern gynecological surgery, experimented on the bodies of enslaved women to develop his techniques for surgical repair of vesicovaginal fistulas (openings or tears between the vagina and rectum or bladder, which can be caused by childbirth). He cruelly experimented on enslaved women, some of whom he bought specifically because they had these fistulas and kept them in his backyard. He performed the surgeries on these women between 1845 and 1849 without the use of anesthesia. He performed as many as 30 surgeries on one particular enslaved woman. The names of these women are largely unknown, with the exceptions of Anarcha, Lucy, and Betsey. The recent awareness of his brutality, and the response to it, has resulted in widespread disavowal and disapproval of Sims as the "father" of modern obstetrics. In 2018, his statue was removed from Central Park in New York City.

By the end of the nineteenth century, birth was medically oriented and largely male dominated. Births still occurred mostly at home but were directed by medical ideas rather than a birthing peoples' intuition and everyday knowledge (Mather 1972; Leighton 1986). New physicians had seen very few normal, physiologic births before they entered practice. Throughout the late nineteenth and early twentieth centuries, interventions increased, often creating new "problems" that called for further interventions. Anesthesia decreased intense contractions but caused breathing difficulties in newborns. Instruments tore birth canal tissue and caused infection. Tissue tears were left torn because suturing could make issues worse. Solutions were usually developed, but not as fast as interventions arose, and caused even more complications.

Post-emancipation, grand midwives were mostly called to attend to birthing people of color but also to white women. They were known as spiritual and traditional healers and care providers, and they tried to maintain the traditional culture of African American community childbirths. Throughout the nineteenth and twentieth centuries, there was still much tradition. Mormon birthing people in Utah relied on midwives until the end of the nineteenth century, when the Mormon Church began sponsoring women to attend women's medical colleges (Rose 1942; Arrington 1976). City and rural immigrant groups also tried keeping tradition as much as possible (Declercq 1985; Ewen 1985; Kobrin 1966). Well into the twentieth century, Black birthing people of the South continued home births, often because they could not afford and did not want medical help, but later they were not even permitted in white hospitals (Devitt 1979; Fraser 1998).

In 1910, 50 percent of all U.S. births were attended by midwives and the other half by general surgeons or gynecologists—not obstetricians (Lee 1996). Physician-attended births were primarily for middle- and upper-class white women. It is noteworthy that more immigrant women of the time began seeking physician attended perinatal care. By the end of the nineteenth century and into the early twentieth century, allopathic physicians—and not "competing sections of healers" vying for "public recognition and support and for the financial rewards of medical practice"—were institutionally represented by the AMA. In the 1920s, however, the American Board of Obstetrics and Gynecology was established to determine the educational qualifications of physicians who were practicing obstetrics and gynecology. The AMA sought professional homogenization and increased standards for medical education (Brickman 1983; Flexner 1910). Meanwhile, the obstetrics specialty struggled to achieve respect and recognition within the medical community. The specialty was thought of as an opening for younger, less experienced physicians to garner skills and later transition to more prestigious and lucrative specialties (Brickman 1983). Borst (1990) notes that for much of the first half of the twentieth century, there was little to no agreement on what constituted an obstetrical specialist.

Along with solidifying the boundaries of the specialty, Borst contends that the specialty, too, "reconceptualized pregnancy as a process with a 'trajectory'; that is, the normative course of pregnancy was understood, but it was also soon to be influenced by systems both within and without the body" (1990, 205). She contends that the physician-patient relationship also shifted with this reconceptualization of pregnancy and childbirth: birth was now something to be managed rather than to be either attended or dominated. All births and all pregnancies were carefully controlled by a process of monitoring. This process of monitoring meant that obstetrics became organized as a hierarchical team (Borst 1990, 206). This hierarchical relationship represents a fundamental difference between physician-managed and midwife-attended care.

Situating pregnancy and childbirth as risky, combined with the sanitary science and germ theory of disease solidified in the late nineteenth century, positioned surgical interventions of high forceps operations and cesarean sections as necessary and safe life-saving procedures (DeLee 1920; Leavitt 1983, 1986). Further, as a result of isolation and hospital intervention practices, people experienced birth as more painful, and drugs were cheaper and deemed more "scientific" than having someone stay with them and provide the "labor support" they have traditionally had. Thus, hospitals and physician-attended births offered analgesic drugs, even "twilight sleep" (the combination of scopolamine and morphine), which midwives were not licensed to provide (Leavitt 1983, 1986; Susie 1988). Collectively, the reconceptualization of pregnancy and birth as requiring risk management, the medical offerings of birth pain relief, and the country's poor maternal and infant mortality statistics of the time were used to argue for greater medical intervention and placed midwives in a vulnerable position. The beginning of the 1920s began a public health solution to the "midwife problem" of the time.

As Ladd-Taylor (1988) reports, "In 1915, approximately six women—eleven black women—died for every 1,000 live births in states where statistics were collected: one hundred infants, and 181 black infants, died for every 1,000 live births" (256–257). Though the greatest contributing factor for the deaths was found to be poverty and not inadequacies in midwifery care, national concerns of maternal and infant mortality put midwives in a rather weakened position. Soon after 1910, progressive, middle-class white women reformers began advocating for the establishment of infant health clinics and pure milk depots and lobbying the government to assume responsibility for child welfare. Their work resulted in the establishment of the United States Children's Bureau in 1912 and the eventual passage of the Sheppard-Towner Maternity and Infancy Protection Act of 1921, which provided federal funding to states to implement maternity and childcare programs. This era introduced state and municipal bureaus of child hygiene, prenatal and child health conferences, educational programs for birth attendants and mothers, and, believing midwives to be responsible for the poor health outcomes, the issuance (or denial) of licenses to midwives. The act began midwifery regulation in the United States, required midwives to be formally supervised, trained, and evaluated by public health nurses.

It is important to note that nurse-midwifery was also established during the 1920s in response to the national concerns of maternal and infant mortality. Following the model of nurse-midwifery in Europe, early nurse-midwives reportedly worked alongside public health nurses funded by the act. This marks the early beginnings of a divided—and racially divided—midwifery community: primarily white nurse-midwives and primarily Black traditional midwives who were descents of grand midwives. Though these trainings were actually not the primary emphasis of the act, the formal supervision, training, and evaluation fundamentally shifted midwifery practice in the United States.

By 1924, 17 states administered classes for midwives (Ladd-Taylor 1988). They were positioned as a "necessary evil," an intermediary until the complete medicalization of pregnancy and childbirth. Sheppard-Towner administrators either infantilized grand midwives ("The negro women, although illiterate and ignorant, are natural nurses and are tractable, teachable, and for the most part, eager to learn the 'white folks' way," said a Mississippi nurse) or demonized them as dangerous, dirty, and "superstitious" practitioners (Darlington 1911; Edgar 1911; Ladd-Taylor 1988; Luke 2018). As a result, functional literacy and participation in medical procedures became a condition for midwifery practice, often leading to the elimination of many older grand midwives (Bonaparte 2015; Logan and Clark 1991; Smith and Holmes 1996). Nurses inspected midwives' bags to ensure that they contained only the supplies legitimated by the Health Department and not substances considered contraband, such as roots, herbs, or homemade salves, all of which were forbidden.

A coalition of medical organizations, chief among them the AMA, fought at the local and national levels against the renewal of the Sheppard-Towner Act in 1927 because they feared the act promoted a socialist agenda toward the universal spread of government control over the budding medical profession (Brickman 1983). After all, great gains were made in the late nineteenth and early twentieth centuries toward professional homogenization with increased standards for entrance into and curriculum in medical schools and greater legitimacy for the obstetrics and gynecology specialty. Prior to this time, the specialty had been little more than an opening wedge through which younger, lesser trained physicians gained more training or the general practitioner sought and won patients (Borst 1990; Flexner 1910). Despite such strong opposition, supporters did succeed in securing federal funding for two more years, but the act was ultimately repealed in 1929. The withdrawal of funds officially restricted the operation of midwife training and regulation but allowed traditional practitioners to continue practicing in remote areas.

By 1935, midwives attended 10 percent of all U.S. births (a 30 percent decrease from 1915). Of those 1935 births, midwives attended only 4.5 percent of white births but 54 percent of nonwhite births (Devitt 1979, 47–48). Still, the practice of midwifery was largely concentrated in the rural South, where the number of Black residents exceeded the number of white residents (Tunc 2010). The Hill-Burton Act of 1946, which provided federal funds for the construction of hospitals in rural areas, was also monumental in shifting birth from the home to hospital, particularly for Black people. For example, in 1935, the percentage of births in hospitals was 27 percent; by 1950, it was 88 percent, and by 1960, it was 96 percent (Devitt 1979, 47).

Beginning in the 1940s and swelling in the 1960s and 1970s was a period of great social and cultural transformation with the civil rights movement, gay rights movement, the feminist movement, the women's health movement, and the home birth movement against the medicalization of pregnancy and birth. As obstetrics and gynecology shifted its focus from the management of the birthing person to monitoring and surveilling the fetus, people began to demand more attention to their needs (Borst 1990). Resisting being treated as a "patient," birthing people desired to be awake, aware, and fully present during birth. The introduction of the Lamaze technique of "childbirth without pain" in the 1940s, Grantly Dick-Read's *Childbirth without Fear* (1944), and Ashley Montagu's (1955) article, "Babies Should Be Born at Home," in the *Ladies' Home Journal* sparked a national dialogue on the increased rates of chemical stimulation of labor, episiotomies, cesarean sections, and the then common practices of not allowing the birthing person's partner or other family in the birthing room and separating them from their newborns immediately after birth.

Yet, it is well documented that women of color reported feeling disconnected from the primarily white feminist home birth and women's health movements for its inattention to issues specific to people of color and birth workers of color (Collins 2000; Craven and Glatzel 2010; Nelson 2003). In many ways, the process of licensing and certifying midwives after the 1960s served to marginalize and exclude practicing midwives, especially in Black, Indigenous, and communities of color. The legitimation of these new midwives as providers often rested on deliberately differentiating themselves as "better educated," more "hygienic," or more "scientific" than midwives of color, while at the same time excluding them from these paths to "legitimate" practice. These new, overwhelmingly white midwives too often failed to acknowledge this history while laying claim to "traditional knowledge," erasing midwives of color from the past and creating an "innocent" present for white-dominant midwifery. The history of direct-entry midwifery that begins in the 1970s with the "white revival" and which describes only the thinnest of top layers on a great foundation of centuries of work by Black, Indigenous, and other people of color is experienced as an act of violence. The effects of this linger today as evidenced by a predominantly white U.S. midwifery workforce (Niles and Drew 2020).

Today midwives in the United States attend approximately 10% of all births. There are three groups of nationally certified midwives in the United States: certified professional midwives (CPM), certified nurse-midwives (CNM), and certified midwives (CM). All three credentials are accredited by the National Commission for Certifying Agencies (NCCA), the accrediting body of the Institute for Credentialing Excellence (ICE).

Certified professional midwives are part of a long and multifaceted tradition of midwifery in the United States, though the credential has a particular history rooted in the home birth movement of the 1970s when birthing people began seeking alternatives to the hospitalization and over-medicalization of birth. The CPM credential was created to define and support these midwives and the first CPM was recognized in 1994; by the end of 2020, approximately 3,839 credentials have been issued. The CPM is the only midwife credential that requires education and training in community settings: homes and birth centers. There are multiple routes to achieving the CPM, including attending one of the 11 schools and programs accredited by the Midwifery Education and Accreditation Council (MEAC), or completing the Portfolio Evaluation Process (PEP), a competency-based apprenticeship with a qualified midwife preceptor. Regardless of the educational route, all CPMs must demonstrate knowledge and skills in all the same competencies and pass the national examination administered by the North American Registry of Midwives (NARM) and recertify every three years. As of January 2021, CPMs are licensed to practice in 34 states and the District of Columbia, with several additional states pursuing licensing in 2021. The National Association of Certified Professional Midwives (NACPM), the professional organization for certified professional midwives, works toward licensure for CPMs in all 50 states and territories and eligibility for third-party reimbursement, including

Medicaid which insures approximately one-half of all birthing families in the United States.

The American College of Nurse-Midwives (ACNM) is the professional association representing certified nurse-midwives (CNMs) and certified midwives (CMs) in the United States. According to the American Midwifery Certification Board, as of August 2020, there were 13,074 CNMs and 117 CMs. The vast majority of midwives in the United States are CNMs. There are 39 accredited nurse midwifery education programs in the country.

Certified nurse-midwives originated in the 1920s and practice primarily in hospitals, with some also practicing in homes, freestanding birth centers or health clinics. A CNM is a Registered Nurse who has met required core competencies and completed a graduate-level midwifery education program. CNMs successfully complete the American Midwifery Certification Board (AMCB) examination to earn the credential and are required to recertify every five years. CNMs are licensed health care providers with prescriptive authority in all 50 states, the District of Columbia and all U.S. territories. CNMs are defined as primary care providers under federal law and care for people throughout their lifetimes. Medicaid, and most private payer reimbursement, is mandatory for CNMs.

Certified midwives are licensed health care providers who have completed the same midwifery education as CNMs and have the same scope of practice. CMs are authorized to practice in six states and have prescriptive authority in two. The first accredited CM education program began in 1996.

In addition to the three national midwife credentials, there are other groups of direct-entry midwives who practice in the United States, including those who identify as traditional midwives. Licensed direct-entry midwives may not be required to hold a national credential by their state licensing laws. All states that license midwives use the NARM national examination as their state examination.

In 2015, the United States Midwifery Education, Regulation, and Association (US MERA) was established. It is a coalition of representatives of national midwifery associations, certifying agencies, and accreditation bodies, representing all credentials, to collaborate toward the collective advancement of midwives and midwifery care in the United States. US MERA established a set of consensus Principles for Model U.S. Midwifery Legislation and Regulation and agreements about educational requirements for midwives. The professional organization for obstetricians and gynecologists, the American College of Obstetricians and Gynecologists, endorsed the US MERA agreements.

Conclusion

In sum, midwifery is an ancient practice, one that brought people together for millennia to sustain the health and well-being of birthing people and their babies, not just to perform operations on the body. It has always been a cultural often spiritual, social, and political practice, as well as one devoted to physiological support, healing, and well-being. How to bring midwives, of all credentials, back in its totality, across racial, ethnic, and class divides, across all 50 states and territories, and to truly be in collaborative practice with obstetricians and other perinatal health providers is an ongoing struggle in the United States.

The history of pregnancy and birth in the United States is of course not only the history of the service providers. What pregnancy and birth mean in society is itself undergoing changes as pregnant, birthing, and childbearing-aged people themselves are resisting obstetric dominance and advocating for person-centered, well-coordinated, respectful, equitable care.

References

Arrington, C. R. 1976. "Pioneer Midwives." In *Mormon Sisters in Early Utah*, edited by C. Bushman, 42–65. Cambridge, MA: Emmaline Press.

Bogdan, J. 1978. "Care or Cure?: Childbirth Practices in Nineteenth Century America." *Feminist Studies* 4: 92–99.

Bonaparte, A. 2015. "Physicians' Discourse for Establishing Authoritative Knowledge in Birthing Work and Reducing the Presence of the Granny Midwife." *Journal of Historical Sociology* 28(2): 166–194.

Borst, C. 1990. "The Professionalization of Obstetrics: Childbirth Becomes a Medical Specialty." In *Women, Health, and Medicine in America: A Historical Handbook*, edited by R. Apple, 197–216. New York: Garland Publishing, Inc.

Brickman, J. P. 1983. "Public Health, Midwives, and Nurses, 1880–1930." In *Nursing History: New Perspectives, New Possibilities*, edited by E. C. Lagemann, 65–88. New York: Teachers College Press.

Briggs, L. 2000. "The Race of Hysteria: 'Overcivilization' and the 'Savage' Woman in Late Nineteenth-Century Obstetrics and Gynecology." *American Quarterly* 52(2): 246–273.

Collins, P. H. 2000. *Black Feminist Thought: Knowledge, Consciousness and the Politics of Empowerment*. New York: Routledge.

Cooper-Owens, D. 2017. *Medical Bondage: Race, Gender, and the Origins of American Gynecology*. Athens: University of Georgia Press.

Craven, C., and M. Glatzel. 2010. "Downplaying Difference: Historical Accounts of African American Midwives and Contemporary Struggles for Midwifery." *Feminist Studies* 366(2): 330–358.

Darlington, T. 1911. "The Present Status of the Midwife." *American Journal of Obstetrics and Diseases in Women and Children* 63: 870–876. https://books.google.com/books?id =TZgxAQAAMAAJ.

Declercq, E. 1985. "The Nature and Style of Practice of Immigrant Midwives in Early Twentieth Century Massachusetts." *Journal of Social History* 19: 118.

DeLee, J. B. 1920. "The Prophylactic Forceps Operation." *American Journal of Obstetrics and Gynecology* 1: 34–44. https://books.google.com/books?id=uHg4AQAAMAAJ.

Devitt, N. 1979. "The Statistical Case for the Elimination of the Midwife: Fact versus Prejudice, 1890–1935, Part 1." *Women and Health* 4(1) (Spring): 79–96.

Donnison, J. 1977. *Midwives and Medical Men: A History of Inter-Professional Social Rivalries and Women's Rights*. New York: Schocken.

Edgar, J. C. 1911. "The Remedy for the Midwife Problem." *American Journal of Obstetrics and Diseases in Women and Children* 63: 881–884. https://books.google.com/books?id =TZgxAQAAMAAJ.

Edwards-Ingram, Y. 2001. "African American Medicine and the Social Relations of Slavery." In *Race and the Archaeology of Identity*, edited by C. E. Orser, 34–53. Salt Lake City: University of Utah Press.

Ewen, E. 1985. *Immigrant Women in the Land of Dollars: Life and Culture on the Lower East Side, 1890–1905*. New York: Monthly Review Press, 131.

Feldstein, R. 2000. "Motherhood in Black and White: Race and Sex in American Liberalism, 1930–1965." Ithaca, NY: Cornell University Press.

Flexner, A. 1910. "Medical Education in the United States and Canada: A Report to the Carnegie Foundation for the Advancement of Teaching." New York: Carnegie Foundation for the Advancement of Teaching.

Fraser, G. J. 1998. *African American Midwifery in the South*. Cambridge, MA: Harvard University Press.

Haynes, R., dir. 2003. *Bringin' in Da Spirit*. Film.

Kapsalis, T. 1997. *Public Privates: Performing Gynecology from Both Ends of the Speculum*. Durham, NC: Duke University Press.

Kobrin, F. 1966. "The American Midwife Controversy: A Crisis of Professionalization." *Bulletin of the History of Medicine* 40: 350–378.

Ladd-Taylor, M. 1988. "'Grannies' and 'Spinsters': Midwife Education under the Sheppard-Towner Act." *Journal of Social History* 22(2): 255–275.

Leavitt, J. W. 1983. "'Science' Enters the Birthing Room: Obstetrics in America since the Eighteenth Century." *Journal of American History* 70(2): 281–304.

Leavitt, J. W. 1986. *Brought to Bed: Childbearing in America 1750 to 1950*. New York: Oxford University Press.

Lee, V. 1996. *Granny Midwives and Black Women Writers: Double-Dutched Readings*. New York: Routledge.

Leighton, A. 1986. *Early American Gardens: For Meate or Medicine*. Amherst: University of Massachusetts Press.

Logan, O. L., and K. Clark. 1991. *Motherwit: An Alabama Midwife's Story*. New York: Penguin Books.

Luke, J. M. 2018. *Delivered by Midwives: African American Midwifery in the Twentieth-Century South*. Jackson: University Press of Mississippi.

Mather, C. 1972. *The Angel of Bethesda: An Essay upon the Common Maladies of Mankind*. Worcester, MA: American Antiquarian Society.

Mongeau, B., H. Smith, and A. Maney. 1961. "The 'Granny' Midwife: Changing Roles and Functions of a Folk Practitioner." *American Journal of Sociology* 66(5): 497–505.

Nelson, J. 2003. *Women of Color and the Reproductive Rights Movement*. New York: New York University Press.

Niles, P. M., and M. Drew. 2020. "Constructing the Modern American Midwife: White Supremacy and White

Feminism Collide." *Nursing Clio.* https://nursingclio.org
/2020/10/22/constructing-the-modern-american-midwife
-white-supremacy-and-white-feminism-collide/.

Norton, M. B. 1996. *Liberty's Daughters: The Revolutionary
Experience of American Women, 1750–1800.* Ithaca, NY:
Cornell University Press.

Owens, D. B. C. 2017. *Medical Bondage: Race, Gender, and
the Origins of American Gynecology.* Athens: University of
Georgia Press.

Rose, B. E. 1942. "Early Utah Medical Practice." *Utah
Historical Quarterly* 10: 14–32.

Schwartz, M. J. 2006. *Birthing a Slave: Motherhood and
Medicine in the Antebellum South.* Cambridge, MA:
Harvard University Press.

Smith, M. C., and L. J. Holmes. 1996. *Listen to Me Good: The
Life Story of an Alabama Midwife.* Columbus: Ohio State
University Press.

Susie, D. A. 1988. *In the Way of Our Grandmothers: A
Cultural View of Twentieth-Century Midwifery in Florida.*
Athens: University of Georgia Press.

Tomes, N. 1997. "Spreading the Germ Theory: Sanitary
Science and Home Economics, 1880–1930." In *Rethinking
Home Economics: Women and the History of a Profession,*
edited by S. Stage and V. Vincenti, 34–54. Ithaca, NY:
Cornell University Press.

Tunc, T. E. 2010. "The Mistress, the Midwife, and the
Medical Doctor: Pregnancy and Childbirth on the
Plantations of the Antebellum American South, 1800–
1860." *Women's History Review* 19(3): 395–419.

White, D. G. 1987. "Ar'n't I a Woman? Female Slaves in the
Plantation South." New York: W. W. Norton, 67–118.

Wilkie, L. A. 2003. *The Archaeology of Mothering: An African-
American Midwife's Tale.* New York: Routledge.

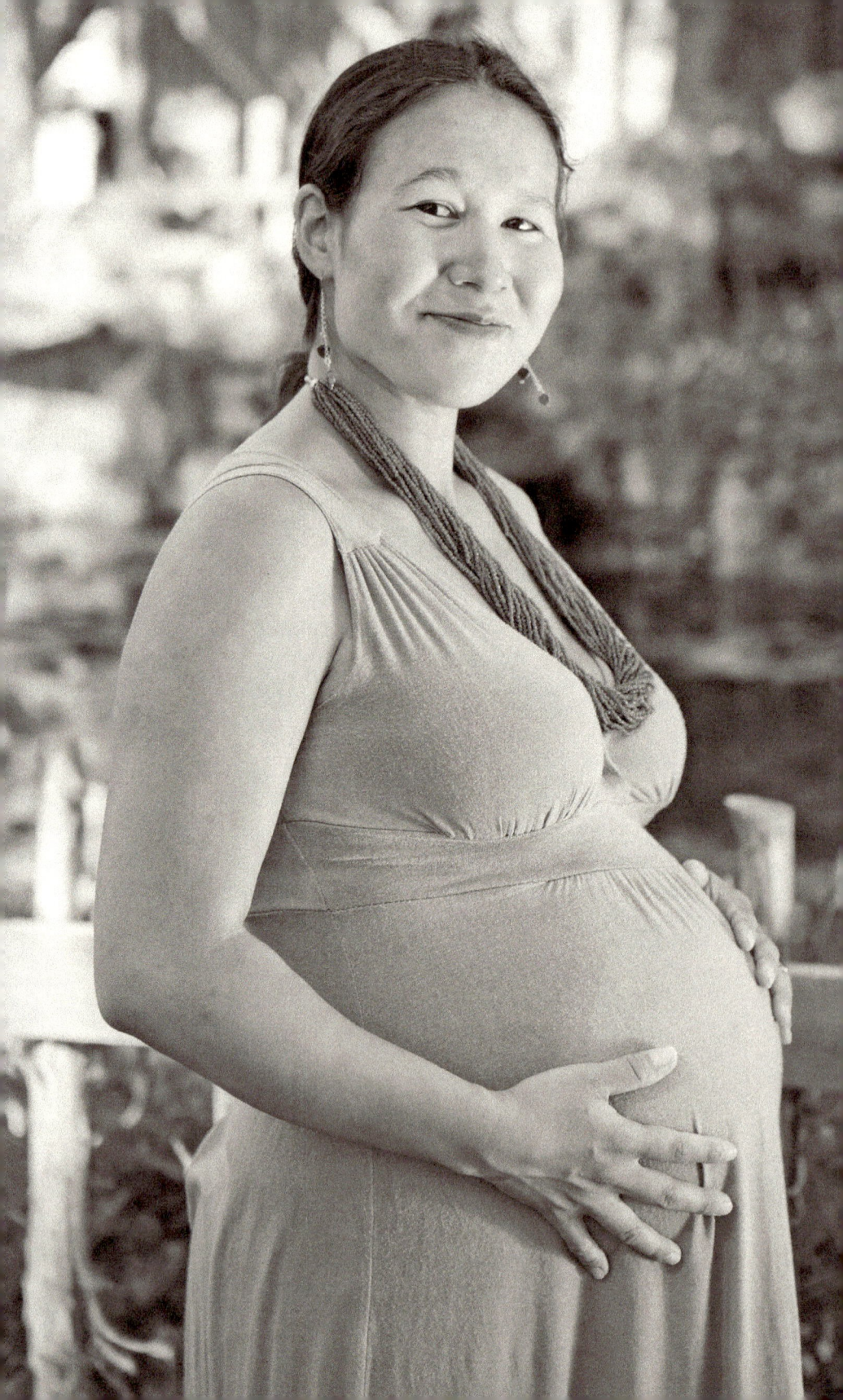

Introduction

This chapter details seven issues that are very important to understanding some of the problems and controversies presented by the U.S. perinatal health care system. Whether in mass media or academic or mainstream literature, these issues, particularly the birthing outcomes and experiences of Indigenous and transgender people, have not gained the urgent attention they deserve. This chapter addresses these issues, along with the professionalization of caring, highlighting media representations of pregnancy and birth, the high costs associated with the perinatal health care system, and the importance of the U.S. census toward allocating more resources. Reproductive Justice is positioned as the most significant framework and practice toward equity in pregnancy and childbirth.

Indigenous Peoples' Birth Outcomes

For many years, Indigenous peoples have been presented with numerous barriers to adequate health care (Novoa and Truschel 2018). Indigenous peoples are more than twice as likely to lack medical insurance. Consequently, they struggle to pay for necessary services and often do not even have access to them (Novoa and Truschel 2018). In many cases, people are so concerned

---

A pregnant person cradling their growing belly. (Mona Makela/Dreams time.com)

with the cost of services that they do not seek medical attention. Additionally, many health care providers put in place to support these communities lack the necessary funding and support to even provide their services properly. For example, Indian Health Services (IHS) is a federal agency responsible for providing health services for Indigenous peoples; however, it is chronically underfunded and lacks emergency services throughout its facilities, making it difficult for people to receive proper medical care, even in life-threatening situations (Novoa and Truschel 2018). It was found that from 2010 to 2012, infants born to Indigenous people faced the risk of infant mortality at a rate of 3.5 times more than white people (Danielson et al. 2018). It is a crisis.

Historical Context

Throughout the 500 years since white colonizers settled in the Americas, there have been many health disparities between Indigenous peoples and other racial/ethnic groups that can be better understood through a deeper historical context. When the IHS was established in 1955, many Indigenous peoples living in rural poverty suffered from tuberculosis and were experiencing an infant mortality rate at four times the national average (Jones 2006). Although improvements have been made over the last 50 years, they have still been suffering more than other groups from tuberculosis, smallpox, alcoholism, and other chronic diseases from the earliest years of colonization all the way until the present day. To better understand this, it is important to review the history of health disparities as well as the social and economic conditions that are contributing factors.

After white colonizers settled in North America mortality rates increased, and every encounter with a new region or population brought on new epidemics, such as smallpox, measles, influenza, and malaria (Jones 2006). While colonists and Indigenous peoples initially experienced the same diseases and natural causes, eventually the colonizers made choices based on local economic and political pressures and had to justify their right to settle on lands that were already inhabited by Indigenous peoples (Jones 2006). By using the fact that Indigenous populations were decreasing faster than their own, the colonizers used health disparities to justify and convince themselves that their mission in America was righteous and led by God to gain political advantage (Jones 2006). In actuality, colonization disrupted Indigenous cultural and social practices that negatively impacted the health of Indigenous peoples. These health disparities, introduced and exacerbated by colonization, are parallel to disparities in wealth and power. The IHS report states that today lower life expectancy and burden of disease exist due to inequities in education and health care systems and the wealth gap (Jones 2006). Awareness of this history, and their current manifestations, is crucial for future research and interventions to directly advance the lives of Indigenous peoples.

Indigenous Health Care

The Changing Woman Initiative is a nonprofit organization with a mission to renew cultural birth knowledge to empower and reclaim Native American sovereignty of women's medicine and life teachings. The founder of this organization is Navajo nurse-midwife Nicolle L. Gonzalez, who for years witnessed Native American women struggle to navigate Western medical health care systems. Assimilation practices, from birth on, impacted Native American families and made it difficult to find ways to bring their loved ones into the world in ceremonial ways that supported their culture and represented their own communities. Since 2015, the Changing Woman Initiative has been growing public awareness of the issues surrounding Native American maternal health and the lack of Native American representation in midwifery throughout the United States, which is often overlooked. The nonprofit also engages with Native American women, doulas, elders, and many more to discuss effective and sustainable ways for these families to access indigenously centered health care with traditional childbirth options for their culture. The Changing Woman Initiative has a vision to honor cultural protocols and offer guidance while honoring language and traditions through compassion and respect for Native American families. In 2012, Nicolle wrote "Making the Case for Indigenous Midwifery" (Gonzalez 2020), which is a statement on the structural issues—colonization, white supremacy, and economic disenfranchisement—impacting the urgent need for more Indigenous midwives serving Indigenous peoples.

Rhonda Lee Grantham is an Indigenous midwife and herbalist from the Cowlitz Nation, a Salish-Sahaptian tribe of Southwest Washington that translates to "Seeker of the Medicine Spirit." For over two decades, she has been actively catching babies and supporting programs within tribal communities, both at home and globally. As the founder of the Center for Indigenous Midwifery, she is guided by her lens as a cultural anthropologist and Native woman, along with her passions for global health, family wellness, and culturally centered care. She is honored to support Indigenous birthkeepers as they share stories, skills, and struggles in dedication of her organization's mission: "Strengthening indigenous communities by honoring, supporting and reclaiming Indigenous midwifery care."

Social Factors Impacting Indigenous Health

In 2010, about 1.7 percent of the U.S. population identified as American Indian and Alaska Native, either alone or in combination with one or more other races (Tribal Public and Environmental Health Think Tank 2018). Throughout the United States, there are 567 federally recognized tribes; however, most Americans remain unaware of the prominent and pressing tribal public and environmental health concerns. The Tribal Public and Environmental Health Think Tank is composed of professionals from diverse backgrounds involving tribal public and environmental health. This think tank has a focus on promoting the voice of the many tribal communities across the United States to raise awareness of and create achievements toward the very unique challenges that these communities face when it comes to public and environmental health. In terms of social awareness, a collective of members from the American Public Health Association has established five social determinants that have affected tribal health and well-being with the hope to educate and inform decision makers and government officials about these issues. These five areas include unsafe and inadequate housing, barriers to educational achievement, persistent generational poverty, deeply rooted historical trauma, and societal and institutional racism and discrimination. It is important to note that in 2020 Deb Haaland (D-NM) was appointed by President-Elect Joe Biden as the first ever Indigenous person to be Interior Secretary, and her appointment was confirmed by the U.S. Senate in March of 2021.

Transgender Peoples' Birth Experiences

In the United States, transgender and gender-variant people experience higher rates of discrimination in housing, education, employment, the criminal justice system, and overall everyday experiences. They experience lower rates of health insurance coverage than the general population (American College of Nurse-Midwives 2012). Additionally, they experience multiple barriers to accessing health care and disproportionately experience negative health outcomes. Unfortunately, gender identity and expression are excluded from federal and most state anti-discriminatory protections.

As the 2012 National Transgender Discrimination Survey demonstrates, experiences of discrimination was a common theme among the 6,450 respondents throughout the United States. However, the report concludes that "the combination of anti-transgender bias and persistent, structural racism was especially devastating. People of color in general fare worse than white participants across the board, with African American transgender respondents faring far worse than all others in most areas examined" (Grant, Mottet, and Tanis 2011, 2).

Another important focus of the lives of transgender individuals involves trans birth and the experiences people have not only with navigating their own bodies and feelings, but also with how they are treated by health care providers and the journey to finding normalcy in their transition to parenthood. Care for pregnant transgender people deserves special attention. When exploring the pregnancy experiences of transmasculine people through interviews, it was found that there was a wide variation of identity expression; some people had a clear preference, such as male, man, female-to-male, transman, transgender man, transmasculine, non-binary, and on the transmasculine spectrum, while others were comfortable with multiple terms for their identity (Hoffkling, Obedin-Maliver, and Sevelius 2017). Many participants had anywhere between one to four pregnancies that resulted in one to three live births (Hoffkling, Obedin-Maliver, and Sevelius 2017). As for social support, there was also a wide variety of feelings and responses from participants. One individual responded to the issue of social support with "I just lost everybody," showing a very isolating experience. Another individual reported an abundance of support, saying, "When it was really obvious that I was a pregnant tranny, I actually received a lot of positive love and affection from queer strangers . . . and I actually had strangers stop and ask if they could hug me and thought that it was beautiful" (Hoffkling, Obedin-Maliver, and Sevelius 2017).

Many transgender people have reported experiences of transphobic health care providers, whether by being addressed by the wrong pronouns or even being laughed at by staff during visits (Hoffkling, Obedin-Maliver, and Sevelius 2017). Many health care providers also often discuss gender identity as if it is the same as sexual identity, completely misunderstanding the identities and lives of their patients. One patient, a transgender person named Braiden Schirtzinger is non-binary and experienced many difficulties while pregnant, ranging from being unable to find nonfeminine maternity clothes to uneasy physician visits and trouble with breastfeeding. They expressed a constant need to correct staff members on their name and pronouns, asking the hospital staff to use the name "B" instead of their legal name "Brittany," but eventually they grew tired of correcting people all the time and also worried that the baby's care might suffer if they spoke up about identifying as non-binary (Schmidt 2019). Braiden also reported experiencing feelings of discomfort when it came to pelvic exams, saying that "being in this pregnant, feminine body felt so wrong" and "wanting to rip their skin off" (Schmidt 2019).

However, many transgender people have also expressed having positive experiences with the health care system. When health care providers use people's pronouns and name, it normalizes and affirms transgender people and their right to respectful care (Hoffkling, Obedin-Maliver, and Sevelius 2017). One patient described the staff as "super-conscientious" about using their appropriate names and pronouns and stated, "They were consulting me before anyone came in the room, using the right pronouns, and they were not weird about it. They didn't ask me any weird questions. It was just unbelievable. I was just kind of blown away at how good they were about it" (Hoffkling, Obedin-Maliver, and Sevelius 2017). Another patient described their experience with staff as valuable and genuine when it came to naming and normalizing their gender by stating, "I walked in and the doctor who I saw, like, the very first one, she was, like, 'look, you're not the first pregnant guy we've had, so don't worry about that.' . . . I just really prefer if health care providers can act as though it's not exceptional or weird to be trans" (Hoffkling, Obedin-Maliver, and Sevelius 2017).

When health care providers normalize transgender identity and experiences, it can help to create rapport with patients and help them to continuously seek care because they feel safe and welcome. As always, positive physiological outcomes will depend on the experience someone has from the beginning to the end of their pregnancy and care that feels inclusive and affirmative (Obedin-Maliver and Makadon 2015).

Respectful, Affirmative Care for LGBTQ People

The World Professional Association for Transgender Health (WPATH) and Gay and Lesbian Medical Association (GLMA) have issued standards of care (Coleman et al. 2012; Gay and Lesbian Medical Association 2006). Furthermore, professional organizations representing perinatal and reproductive health care providers in the United States have established organizational values or commitments or issued briefs affirming the rights of LGBTQ people; a commitment to compassionate, affirming, and equitable care free of discrimination, violence, homophobia, biphobia, and transphobia; and, a commitment to gender-inclusive language (American College of Obstetricians and Gynecologists 2012; Black Mamas Matter Alliance 2021; International Confederation of Midwives 2017; Midwives Alliance North America 2014; National Association of Certified Professional Midwives 2014; National Association to Advance Black Birth 2018; Maura 2019). We highlight the mission of Birth for Everybody (n.d.), which well captures the importance of such commitments:

> We honor and uphold the right to self-determination and bodily autonomy for all people. We believe that as midwives, our purpose is to support parents and babies throughout the childbearing year, taking into account the unique physiological, psychological, and social well-being and needs of each client. It is our work to provide individualized education and counseling, as well as client-centered prenatal, intrapartum, and postpartum care. We understand the importance of providing compassionate,

holistic, and culturally sensitive midwifery care, and we strive towards making the Midwives Model of Care™ accessible for every person and family who seeks it, regardless of race, ethnicity, religion, ability, sexual orientation, gender identity or gender expression. We acknowledge the disproportionate effects of transphobia on those with other marginalized identities such as being a person of color, low-income or disabled. Many racial health disparities that concern midwives and impact our communities are experienced in greater numbers by people who are both Black and transgender. These lives especially are in need of the kind of respectful, compassionate, and individualized care midwives can offer. We assert that we can honor the power of all women while at the same time extending this reverence to all people who are pregnant and giving birth, and that to do so is in full alignment with the heart of midwifery.

Recruiting and retaining gender-variant and LGBTQ people must also be an essential component of this work as they are currently underrepresented perinatal health care providers. A 2018 American Association of Medical Colleges report found that less than 1 percent of matriculated students identify as gender non-binary or transgender. More research is needed to determine the percentage of LGBTQ providers in order to best meet the needs of pregnant and birthing people.

The annotated bibliography presented in chapter 6 includes many resources by and for LGBTQ pregnant and birthing people and families.

Professionalization of Caring

One of the important contributions of feminist sociology was to point out how much of the work that goes on in any society, and specifically in a capitalist society such as ours, occurs outside of formal and public paid settings. For a worker to show up at work, someone had to have carried, birthed, tended to, and raised that worker; someone had to provide them food, clothing, and care of their children, the next generation of workers. This work, often called *invisible labor* or *invisible work* was typically performed by women, especially women of color (Daniels 1987). During World War II, when women were brought into the workforce to substitute for the men who had been moved to the front lines, factories had to provide breakfasts, lunches, and sometimes dinners to take home; laundering services for uniforms; and childcare. When the war was over and the women were fired and sent back home, the factories stopped providing those things.

As women moved back into the workforce in large numbers through the 1970s and onward, including women with young children, issues of childcare and other traditional invisible labor began to reenter public discussion. As sociologist Arlie Russell Hochschild pointed out, more and more of what had been understood as private and family life has been "outsourced," sold as consumable services (Hochschild 2012).

When work is done at home, there may be powerful societal and cultural expectations about how it is to be done, what constitutes doing it right or not, but these remain in the informal sector. When work is hired out, it becomes *professionalized*, with external standards. When, for example, a parent or a sibling or a grandparent is teaching a three-year-old how to read or how to name the animals in a picture book, there is no formal oversight. When that same activity is taking place in a preschool setting, the person doing the work is expected to be specifically trained, to have shared understandings of age-appropriate knowledge, and to have very specific skills.

As American society has moved more and more from the manufacturing of objects as our economic base to what is called the *service economy*, more and more tasks move into that realm of professionalized work. And so it is with much of the work surrounding the care of pregnancy, birth, and early parenthood.

These services, generally understood to be part of health services, moved from family and community into centralized medical services. Birth itself became hospital-based. But the basic care of pregnant and postpartum people and babies also moved into medical management. In that medical system, the issues of specific training, shared understanding and knowledge, and specific skills become key. There are of course the standardized medical school curricula, but nursing care at all different levels has also been standardized. A pregnant person is expected to see medical professionals for standardized testing and examination at regular intervals through the pregnancy; a baby is brought into pediatric offices for those same kinds of testing and examinations as well as for vaccinations.

With standardized technical services, the more personal, individualized care tends to be separated out and lost. In ordinary English language, we talk about "medical care," but having your blood pressure checked or being weighed or prescribed drugs are not what we usually think of as caregiving or caring work. Within the medical settings, the more standardized services tend to move down the occupational hierarchy and be done in more and more tightly controlled and standardized ways. But clearly people in pregnancy, people in labor, and people caring for newborn babies require some emotional support and individualized attention. This work historically moved along gender and race lines: white male physicians provided the technical services, and female nurses, usually white, provided the care. Over time, the gendered differences have shifted somewhat, but there are clear racial and gender divisions to be found in American medical systems. But focusing on the division between technical and caring services, greater focus on technical care and greater valuing of technical skills have meant that caring becomes devalued. We used to think of nursing as specifically caring and nurturing work. Physicians came and did the surgery or amputation or whatever work on the body, and nurses tended to the personal. Over time, nurses and those lower down an elitist hierarchy, such as the aides of various forms, have had their work increasingly professionalized; the technical skills are acknowledged, and the caring becomes a kind of invisible labor and is not necessarily provided at all.

In the arena of birth, the various waves of social movements to improve birth care, from the "prepared" birth movement of the post–World War II era to the home birth movement of the 1970s to Reproductive Justice movement (see below), have all focused on some aspect of care work. In the 1950s, the industrialization of birth left people alone in labor, with no emotional or support care at all. That first movement was to permit someone they know, a partner most commonly, to be with them in labor and to be there for the birth as well. That person could help the birthing person do calming breathing exercises, talk to them, and hold their hand. They provided no "technical skills" or services and could not so much as touch the person without medical approval. The accompanying caregiver stood at their head while the physicians and medical personnel were at the other end of the delivery table, extracting the fetus.

In the home birth movement, one key idea was that if one properly met the social and emotional needs of the birthing person and dealt with birth in a physiologically helpful way, the technical care became less central and less urgent. For a birthing person who is physically and emotionally comfortable, birth is itself safer. Sitting or squatting upright or lying on their side rather than strapped on their back, for example, the person could push the baby out. Midwives were valued for their technical skills, most especially "if something goes wrong" or if birth does not come readily and unassisted. But midwives were also valued for their skills in caring—the idea that *caring* can also involve skills. In the popular discussion, the idea that took hold was that if birth was "natural," no skills were needed. That was not what proponents of either the 1950s prepared birth or the home birth movement midwives were claiming. But it was an idea that fit in with the deep medicalization of birth, the idea that physicians "deliver" babies. And it fits with the larger cultural notion of skilled technical work and the invisible labor of caring. In this cultural context, one solution offered is to professionalize the caring itself, to focus on caring as something that can be standardized, meaning work for which people can be trained and evaluated.

Current movements, focusing on how institutional racism produces racial-ethnic disparities in infant and maternal morbidity and mortality rates, have in some ways accepted this division of childbirth services into the professional, technical medical services and the caring work. The physicians and nurses provide the technical services, and other providers are generally expected to provide the caring services. But if those people are not of the racial-ethnic group of the people being cared for, the likelihood of racism affecting one's experiences and outcomes are increased. In the greater scheme of things, there should be a representative assortment of workers at all levels. In the world we are living in, the higher one goes up the occupational ladder, the more white the providers.

One solution has been to hire care workers for pregnancy and labor support. People to aid pregnant people in solidifying a birth plan that identifies their wants, needs, and desires; encourage laboring and birthing people and assess their needs; and communicate that to the providers to assure respectful and caring attention. The model that the movement has drawn on is the doula. The word *doula* comes from the Greek word for "maidservant." Anthropologist Dana Raphael (1973) used the word *doula* in the area of birth when she wrote about the necessity of "mothering the mother," particularly during postpartum, to increase the odds of successful breastfeeding. Raphael noted that most cultures provided some of that kind of doula care, someone, usually but not necessarily a woman, often but not always with much experience, whose role was to care for the mother. It was the presence of a caring person attending to the mother that was essential (Raphael 1973, 141).

People in the medical world took the term *doula* and moved it out of the familial, communal realm and used it for "an experienced labor companion who provides the woman and her husband or partner with emotional and physical support throughout the entire labor and delivery, and to some extent afterward" (Klaus, Kennel, and Klaus 2002). The role thus moved beyond familial and personal relationships. This is a prime example of the professionalization of caring.

Several key challenges accompany this professionalization. One issue is how to standardize individualized care. It seems almost a contradiction in terms that standardized care and skills will meet individual needs. American society does do this with other areas of personal care; psychological counseling is perhaps a prime example. A highly trained professional can distinguish individual needs and meet those needs appropriately. Is labor care comparable? Can a well-trained, experienced professionalized carer recognize the very different needs of different people in labor? Most of us know that some people want more holding and touching, and some want less; some people express pain loudly and vocally, others quietly. One can read the face of someone you know very well but read someone you do not know less effectively. In a therapeutic relationship with a psychotherapist, there will be hours of initial meetings and exploration. For birth care, there may be some meetings ahead of time, or a doula might be assigned late in pregnancy or even at birth. The doula may not have gone through painful, frightening experiences with the pregnant person repeatedly before the labor—which itself can be both painful and frightening.

The other and perhaps more fundamental problem is precisely the problem that occurred in the early childbirth movement: the separation of caring from the more highly valued technical care means that the people doing the technical care hold the power. The doula, like the partner in the 1950s, can be supportive and caring, and unlike the partner, the doula probably knows more about birth and the hospital system—but neither has systematic power. If the medical provider wants to do a cesarean section, for example, or move a newborn into an intensive care nursery, the person hired for caring is not empowered by the system to stop that.

The popular discourse often talks about "midwives and doulas," as if they are essentially the same thing, caring providers of emotional support for birth. Obstetric dominance has separated technical services from care work. The devaluing of caring has also contributed to conflating two very different occupational roles. Midwives are technically trained and educated as primary perinatal health care providers. Their skills directly challenge obstetric dominance. Doulas, too, are trained, though their competencies are obviously different, and the training is much shorter. The Doulas of North America (DONA) training program is 16 hours, for example, while Ancient Song Doulas Services offers a 3-day Full Spectrum Doulas Training Program and a 7-Week Full Spectrum Labor and Postpartum Training. The work of both midwives and doulas are needed. Yet, it is obstetric dominance and the medicalization of pregnancy and birth, contributing to poor outcomes detailed in chapter 5, that continues to demand resistance.

Media Representations of Pregnancy and Birth

The average American watches more than 5 hours of live television per day (Hinckley 2014). People between the ages of 2 and 11 spend approximately 24 hours per week watching television, followed by about 21 hours for those ages 12 to 17, 23 hours for those 18 to 24, 28 hours for those 25 to 34, 34 hours for those 35 to 49, 44 hours for those 50 to 64, and more than 50 hours for those 65 and older (Hinckley 2014). Additionally, the average American spends another 32 minutes per day on time-shifted television, one hour on the internet or computer, over an hour on a smartphone, and almost three hours listening to music (Hinckley 2014). African Americans spend an average of 218 hours per month watching television, while whites spend about 156 hours, Hispanics spend about 124 hours, and Asian Americans spend about 93 hours (Hinckley 2014). Overall, this report shows a great deal of screen time for those of younger ages, a slight drop during the teenage years when people are more likely to have outside interests, and then a continuous rise in television viewing for the remainder of our lives, especially with Americans having the ever-growing world of technology at their fingertips through the use of smartphones, tablets, and other internet and streaming devices.

Considerable debate surrounds the influence that media can have on first-time pregnant people (Luce et al. 2016). Six companies Comcast/NBC Universal, News Corporation, the Walt Disney Company, Viacom/CBS Corporation, Time Warner, and Sony Corporation of America own approximately 90 percent of the U.S. mass media market, wielding immense power in the creation and reflection of our culture, that is, in the dismantling or perpetuation of images (Lutz 2012). Television is one of the primary sources of health information for people throughout the United States, and two-thirds of expectant people report watching reality television programs surrounding the topic of birth (Vitek and Ward 2019). Many people watch these television programs to learn and to attempt to understand the birth experience because it may be their only opportunity to witness the process before experiencing it themselves. Yet, reality television is hypersensationalized and consistently portrays birth as risky, dangerous, unpredictable, painful, and requiring medical intervention (Luce et al. 2016). The absence of portrayals of normal physiologic birth has reportedly led to heightened anxieties and fears among pregnant people and an overall increase in the anticipation of negative, even life-threatening, outcomes (Luce et al. 2016).

These exposures to unrealistic depictions of birth often diminish birth self-efficacy, or people's confidence in their body's ability to handle birth (Vitek and Ward 2019). The technocratic model of birth frames the childbearing body as weak, unpredictable, and susceptible to "malfunction" during birth (Vitek and Ward 2019). Again, this model is responsible for increasingly unnecessary medical interventions, as evidenced by the astronomically high cesarean and morbidity and mortality rates in the United States. It is actually the increased likelihood of unnecessary medical intervention that is the real risk.

In 2008, Alicia VandeVusse presented a paper, "*A Baby Story* as a Source of Information about Childbirth: The Messages and Their Implications," at the American Sociological Association Annual Conference. Premiering in 1998, *A Baby Story* is a popular reality television show that follows women and couples during the late stages of pregnancy and childbirth. VandeVusse analyzed 40 episodes of the show and identified all discussions of medical interventions, previous births, and expectations for birth. Noting that the sampled episodes did portray a higher proportion of midwife-attended and home births and a lower proportion of cesarean sections than the current national averages, much of the show's programming centered less on birth options and more on pain; yet, the discussions of medical interventions and other birth experiences were largely limited to commentaries regarding birthing people's feelings toward epidurals, a topic closely related to the fear of pain and the desire (or not) for pain relief. By emphasizing the fear of pain and extolling the effectiveness of epidurals, many episodes portrayed epidurals as a panacea for labor issues. At the same time, many episodes treated epidurals and other medical interventions as matters of due course, noting their occurrence with a brief comment or not at all.

The lack of clear information regarding interventions and decision making during birth has an impact on what viewers can pick up by watching the show. Some interventions are never explicitly discussed or shown, and it is not clarified whether the reason for this omission is the subject's perceived inappropriateness for public display, a failure to make interesting television, a lack of time in the show, a combination of these, or something else entirely. However, the result is a narrow picture of what birth is like for the majority of birthing people today. Because birth options are not clearly stated and interventions often occur off camera or without comment, in these episodes, the medicalized version of birth is enshrined as the normal course of events, and alternatives are recognized in the small subset of episodes in which midwives are the primary birth attendants or the birthing people are particularly "stubborn." In addition, structural aspects of the show (i.e., the brevity of the depicted labors and the discreet camera angles) may give people unrealistic expectations for birth. Such a narrow focus on pain is a missed opportunity for larger discussions of birthing options and decision making, thus further dominating the medical model and obscuring understandings of choice and power.

Further analysis has pointed to the ways in which fictionalized representations of midwifery in prime-time television represented midwives as callous in terms of their personalities. That is, the contemporary stigmatizing represented in these shows reduced midwives to mean and uncaring who in no way enhanced the birth experience and actually detracted from a better birth experience by not providing drugs for pain relief. In the episodes of *Dharma & Greg*, *Gilmore Girls*, and *Girlfriends* (the only show of these three starring African American characters), the author found that midwives were no longer overtly demonized as ignorant and meandering, as in decades before, but were characterized as "controlling bitches," forcing people to suffer in pain, the clear opposite of that typified in the Midwives Model of Care. The people who choose midwives, then, are considered crazy, fringe lunatics who are naturally unsupported by their partners and family members for their seemingly irrational choice to birth with a midwife.

In a discussion of the ways in which humorous shows offer an opportunity for negotiation of controversial social issues, Kline (2007) analyzes the effects of framing on such representation. She states that "fictionalized accounts of social issues function as a means of public argumentation by framing and defining representations to reveal an attitude toward and, thus, implicitly proposing a solution to a given social concern. In other words, frames serve as responses to disruption of the social order and framing choices represent a rhetor's attempt to re-form or repair social fractures." In this way, midwifery plot lines, Kline teaches, are situated in a burlesque frame in which the villain (here midwife) behaves so heinously that they are readily identified as the antagonist who must be banished and is most often ridiculed and turned into a caricature. While too much weight may be given to humorous shows' ability to propose a solution or repair social fractures, they do, however, start a conversation, creating entryways for new possibilities (one need only consider popular prime-time television shows such as *Will & Grace*, *Glee*, and *Modern Family* and their impact on public perceptions of homosexuality). The burlesque framing of midwifery plot lines does not serve to fairly introduce midwifery or the Midwives Model of Care to mainstream audiences. Instead, as VandeVusse found with reality television, it serves to solidify the dominant medical model of birth, which is problematic given the worsening outcomes. Still, arguably more so than birth outcome data, such images are embedded more so in our culture and on our psyches.

Another concern regarding media portrayals of childbirth is the glamorization of pregnancy. Many birthing people report that their exposure to unrealistic images and messages often leads to negative emotions, including self-consciousness about their bodies, depression, frustration, and a feeling of hopelessness because of societal pressures to immediately and miraculously return to their pre-pregnancy weight (Asian News International 2017). Many birthing people feel that media portrayals of pregnant and postpartum bodies are idealistic and far removed from the average person's actual experience (Asian News International 2017). The idea of celebrities losing all of their baby weight in record time that is captured through the media also sets unrealistic expectations and does not take into account how much time is needed for physical healing or the stress that can come with taking care of a newborn baby. The annotated bibliography presented in chapter 6 includes many resources on media portrayals of pregnancy and birth. Still, further research is needed to understand how media images—especially social media images—impact people's perceptions of pregnancy and birth and birth providers, especially midwives.

Perinatal Health Care System Cost

This section has been adapted with permission from NACPM's 2016 Bundled Payment Proposal (http://nacpm.org/wp-content/uploads/2016/01/1.15.16-NACPM-Bundled-Payment-Proposal.pdf).

Perinatal health care is a key driver of health care costs. Care of childbearing people and newborns is the number one reason for hospitalization in the United States; in 2009, maternal and newborn hospital admissions accounted for 23 percent of all hospital stays (Wier et al. 2011). Total estimated charges for hospital alone, not including professional fees (e.g., obstetrician, midwife, anesthesiologist, pediatrician), were about $126 billion in 2013. Hospital maternal and newborn charges increased by 90 percent in the decade from 2003 to 2013, while the total number of births decreased by 4 percent over the same period (Agency for Healthcare Research and Quality 2009). Medicaid is the largest payer for maternal and newborn care it paid for 45 percent of all maternal hospital stays in the United States in 2009 (Wier et al. 2011).

Perinatal health care in the United States is characterized by overuse of expensive technologies and underuse of many beneficial forms of care. For example, cesarean section has become the most commonly performed surgery in the United States (Wier et al. 2011). The overall cesarean delivery rate in the United States has increased by over 60 percent from the late 1990s through the mid-2000s. According to *National Vital Statistics Reports*, the cesarean delivery rate increased from 31.9 percent in 2016 to 32.0 percent in 2017 (Martin et al. 2017, 6). For most low-risk pregnancies, cesarean birth poses a greater risk of complications and death than vaginal birth, and the risk of certain complications, such as placental abnormalities, increases with each cesarean (Cho and Norman 2013; Gregory et al. 2012; Clark and Silver 2011). Overwhelming evidence shows that having a vaginal birth after a cesarean (VBAC) would be an appropriate option for a very large proportion of people with a cesarean history (Guise et al. 2010). According to *National Vital Statistics Reports*, in 2017, 12.8 percent of birthing people with a previous cesarean delivered vaginally, an increase from 12.4 percent in the previous year (Martin et al. 2017, 6).

Other underused forms of care with clear support from rigorous systematic reviews include smoking cessation intervention in pregnancy, external version to turn fetuses that are not headfirst near the end of pregnancy, doula care/continuous support during labor, drug-free measures for comfort and progress in labor, ambulation and upright positioning in labor, intermittent auscultation for fetal monitoring, early skin-to-skin contact, and lactation support.

In the United States, 98.8 percent of births occur in hospitals, and 0.3 percent of births take place in birthing centers (Dekker 2013). We increasingly understand that birth in community settings—birth centers and home births—are beneficial and less expensive alternatives to hospital births for lower-risk people (Shah 2015; Hill et al. 2014). Further, even if the actual birth occurs in the hospital, cesarean section rates and the cost of vaginal birth are lower if a midwife or birth center has managed the prenatal care and manages the birth in the hospital (Howell et al. 2014; Johantgen et al. 2012). A meta-analysis comparing studies of home and hospital births (Wax et al. 2010) found that the following outcomes favored home: reduced preterm birth and low birth weight; reduced use of epidural, electronic fetal monitoring, episiotomy, operative vaginal birth, and cesarean birth; and reduced lacerations (any perineal, third- and fourth-degree perineal, vaginal), infection, postpartum bleeding/hemorrhage, and retained placenta. The study found no difference in perinatal mortality, newborn ventilation, cord prolapse, or large gestation babies. The home birth studies reported more babies born at post-term. The sole outcome of concern in the home birth group was greater neonatal death, which is a controversial result for many reasons; for example, some included studies could not exclude higher-risk unplanned out-of-hospital births, and there was a small number of home birth babies (16,500) for the neonatal mortality comparison versus the twentyfold greater number of home birth babies included in the no-difference comparison for perinatal mortality (331,666) (Michal et al. 2011). A subsequent report of nearly 17,000 who planned home births reported favorable results congruent with the 2010 meta-analysis (Cheyney et al. 2014).

A 2007 study in Washington State found that community-based births (at home or in freestanding birth centers) attended by certified professional midwives (CPMs) resulted in fewer low birth weight babies and much lower cesarean section rates while delivering substantial savings to the state budget (Health Management Associates 2007). A more recent study examined whether birth center care would reduce Medicaid costs and found an average savings of $1,163 per birth, or $11.6 million in savings per 10,000 births per year (Howell et al. 2014). This same study found that in the District of Columbia, the difference in Medicaid costs between a vaginal birth in a birth center and one in a hospital was $3,281 ($6,468 versus $3,187 in 2008). A national study of average total payments over the full episode of perinatal care in 2010 documented significant costs for both commercially insured people and babies ($18,329 for vaginal and $27,866 for cesarean births) and for those covered by Medicaid ($9,131 for vaginal and $13,590 for cesarean births) (Truven Health Analytics 2013).

Furthermore, researchers at the University of Washington studied 657,061 Americans with employer-based insurance plans who gave birth between 2008 and 2015. The Affordable Care Act (ACA) requires employer-based insurance plans to cover perinatal services, but plans are allowed to impose cost sharing, such as copayments and deductibles, for these services. Analyzing insurance claims during the year prior to delivery, during the delivery itself, and for three month after, the researchers found that more and more American birthing people are on plans with high deductibles in recent years, as employers have sought to shift health care costs onto employees: "The percentage of women with deductibles rose from about 69 percent to about 87 percent in the seven-year time period. Women paid a greater share—about 7 percent more—of their childbirth expenses are a result" (Khazan 2020, 2). Again, given that childbirth is the number one reason for hospitalization among American birthing people and that perinatal care represents the most expensive hospital-billed condition billed to commercial insurers, the need to address the cost of care is urgent.

A large proportion of people who currently give birth in hospitals would meet criteria for giving birth in community settings and, further, are interested in or open to considering those settings (Declercq 2012). If only a small percent of those 98.8 percent of U.S. births in hospitals were shifted to community settings, savings and health benefits could be significant. The American Public Health Association (APHA) recommends midwives as the most appropriate and cost-effective providers for the majority of women (American Public Health Association 2000). Although most people give birth in hospitals attended by obstetricians, a growing number are choosing to give birth at birth centers or at home attended by certified nurse-midwives (CNMs) or certified professional midwives (CPMs). In 2013, more than 56,000 births took place outside the hospital (Martin et al. 2015).

With over $126 billion in hospital charges alone at stake—one of the largest single costs in our health care system—a model that encourages broader choice for people and their families could save significant dollars for payers, purchasers, taxpayers, and consumers in out-of-pocket costs. If the outcomes are comparable and often better and the costs are less, why are so few people being encouraged to use these other options? The answer lies in the limited coverage for these providers and settings, inadequate knowledge of the choices available, and a lack of incentives for using them. Medicaid and private coverage remains very limited for these other options—either they are not covered at all or are covered at very low reimbursement levels. With the shift toward managed care in the Medicaid program, this issue has grown even more problematic.

Even if all the options are covered, birthing people are typically on their own in choosing their providers, with no real discussion of site of care options. Further, the payment system rewards the providers who deliver the higher-tech hospital experience with higher payments. In fact, the level of payment for the nonhospital setting and midwives is often so low that it limits the supply of these practitioners, who struggle to continue their practices.

But even more worrisome is that in a time when the health care system is working to transform into a system that rewards value, the incentives for birth encourage the use of higher-cost cesarean sections and higher-cost hospital births versus birth centers or home births and higher-cost providers—physicians rather than midwives. The evidence strongly suggests that a healthy person with an uncomplicated pregnancy and a single full-term baby in a head-down position can safely be managed in a community birth setting. Yet, when only 0.3 percent of births occur in these settings, the nation is not doing its best to create value for pregnant people and their families (Dekker 2013).

An additional concern is the limited information that pregnant people can find in provider directories and implications for their choices. While they can generally search for obstetrician-gynecologists, many of those practitioners have retired from providing perinatal care, may have limits on accepting new patients, or may not be a good match for the person seeking care. Further, a very large proportion of U.S. counties have no currently practicing obstetrical provider (Rayburn 2011). Typically, provider directories do not identify available midwives and family physicians as able to provide perinatal care.

See Chapter 5 for more comprehensive information on the data presented in this section.

Every Baby Counts

As if counting every single person in the U.S. census was not difficult enough, counting every infant and toddler throughout the country adds an even greater challenge. Parents and adults with young children are often unaware that they must include all children who live with them, even if the living situation is part-time. According to the U.S. Census Bureau, in 2010, nearly one million children were not counted in the census, and the largest group of undercounted people are those under the age of five. Missing children in the census are due to a number of factors, such as adults simply not returning the questionnaire, leaving off children who only live with them temporarily, and, most commonly, misreporting children from "complex households," or those with multigenerational or blended families. This is also an issue in households with limited English-speaking skills or those living in poverty. Many families are also often afraid to count children due to immigration status; however, responses to the 2020 census are protected by law, completely confidential, and cannot be shared with landlords, law enforcement, or immigration agencies.

Not counting newborns and young children in the census is a large-scale issue that can impact families, communities, and neighborhoods for years to come. Local, state, and federal lawmakers use the census population statistics to determine how to spend billions of dollars in federal and state funds for the next ten years, and a large portion of that money funds programs that directly affect children. These programs range from nutrition assistance, Head Start, special education, foster care, Medicaid, and children's insurance and housing assistance. Having an accurate count of all children living within the population not only affects decisions made at the state level but at the local level as well. Many local decisions, such as building new schools, libraries, or hospitals, are driven by community population statistics. If all the children in a community are not accounted for, this leads to many children and families not receiving the proper funds and resources to succeed in many crucial areas, such as education, health, and overall well-being and quality of life. While this task is extremely challenging, the Census Bureau is increasing its efforts to inform and educate the public on including children in the census if they live and sleep in the home for most of the time and how crucial this is for the improvement of the lives of children and families not only in underserved communities but also the entire U.S. population.

Reproductive Justice

Reproductive Justice is "the human right to maintain personal bodily autonomy, have children, not have children, and parent the children we have in safe and sustainable communities" (https://www.sistersong.net/reproductive-justice; Ross and Solinger 2017). SisterSong is a collective led by people of color that provides an important history to Reproductive Justice as both a framework and as a practice:

> Indigenous women, women of color, and trans* people have always fought for Reproductive Justice, but the term was invented in 1994. Right before attending the International Conference on Population and Development in Cairo, where the entire world agreed that the individual right to plan your own family must be central to global development, a group of black women gathered in Chicago in June of 1994. They recognized that the women's rights movement, led by and representing middle class and wealthy white women, could not defend the needs of women of color and other marginalized women and trans* people. We needed to lead our own national movement to uplift the needs of the most marginalized women, families, and communities.

> Reproductive Justice demands an analysis and dismantling of power systems such as white supremacy, racism, and capitalism

that disproportionally impact the lives and birthing experiences of Black, Indigenous, and people of color. It demands attention to social determinants of health such as economic and housing security and more upstream structural determinants of health such as paid family leave, health insurance coverage, and scope and investment in communities (Crear-Perry et al. 2020). Reproductive Justice demands a perinatal health care workforce that represents the diverse U.S. population. It puts the person back in the body, not simply dwindling people down to data outcomes and disparities, like those you will be introduced to in chapter 5. Reproductive Justice is the vehicle for better and more equitable outcomes, experiences, and policies.

Conclusion

Indigenous people's birth outcomes reflect a legacy of colonization that is still impacting the community more generally, particularly in birth and birth outcomes. Addressing this issue requires a national willingness to not only acknowledge this history but also to have substantive social and economic legislation and policy to provide quality resources and do no further harm, including respecting tribal lands and tribal sovereignty.

While various maternity care providers and professional organizations have documented commitments to best serving and supporting the LGBTQ community in pregnancy and birth, more attention must be paid to listening to their experiences. Much can be gained from more in-depth qualitative analyses of experience because it should inform policies and practices to address some of the issues raised herein.

We recognize that it takes time to right wrongs and better understand the experiences of communities that have long been underserved. There must be a truth-telling and reconciliation before justice can truly be achieved. It is possible. There *are* ways to address the astronomical costs (and poor outcomes) associated with birth, as demonstrated herein. There *are* ways to address media representations of pregnancy and childbirth—show normal physiological birth; show midwives in homes, birthing centers, and hospitals; show perinatal health workers and other birth workers, such as doulas, lactation consultants, and nutritionists. And, to better allocate resources that families, communities, and neighborhoods so desperately need, make every person count by completing the U.S. census. Yet, absolutely none of this is possible without Reproductive Justice.

References

Agency for Healthcare Research and Quality. 2009. "HCUPnet: Healthcare Cost and Utilization Project." https://hcupnet.ahrq.gov/#setup.

American College of Nurse-Midwives. 2012. "Position Statement: Transgender/Transsexual/Gender Variant Health Care." http://www.midwife.org/acnm/files /ACNMLibraryData/UPLOADFILENAME /000000000278/Transgender%20Gender%20Variant %20Position%20Statement%20December%202012.pdf.

American College of Obstetricians and Gynecologists. 2012. "Health Care for Lesbians and Bisexual Women." ACOG Committee Opinion Number 25: Health Care for Underserved Women.

American Public Health Association. 2000. "Supporting Access to Midwifery Services in the United States." https:// www.apha.org/policies-and-advocacy/public-health-policy -statements/policy-database/2014/07/29/08/22/supporting -access-to-midwifery-services-in-the-united-states-position -paper#:~:text=The%20American%20Public%20 Health%20Association,subsequent%20improvement%20 of%20birth%20outcomes.

Asian News International. 2017. "Unrealistic Media Portrayals of Pregnancy Put Women at Risk." https://www .hindustantimes.com/more-lifestyle/media-unrealistically

-portrays-the-glamour-of-pregnancy-puts-women-at-risk
/story-1vhSM7IOI8ewmshitsGDBP.html.

Association of American Medical Colleges. 2018.
"Matriculating Student Questionnaire." https://www.aamc
.org/media/9641/download.

Birth for Everybody. n.d. "Our Mission." Accessed January
21, 2021. http://www.birthforeverybody.org/.

Black Mamas Matter Alliance. 2021. "Values." https://
blackmamasmatter.org/values/.

Cheyney, M., M. Bovbjerg, C. Everson, W. Gordon, D.
Hannibal, and S. Vedam. 2014. "Outcomes of Care for
16,484 Planned Home Births in the United States: The
Midwives Alliance of North America Statistics Project,
2004–2009." *Journal of Midwifery and Women's Health*
59(1): 17–27.

Cho, C. E., and M. Norman. 2013. "Cesarean Section and
Development of the Immune System in the Offspring."
American Journal of Obstetrics and Gynecology 208(4):
249–254.

Clark, E. A., and R. M. Silver. 2011. "Long-Term Maternal
Morbidity Associated with Repeat Cesarean Delivery."
American Journal of Obstetrics and Gynecology 205(6):
S2–10.

Coleman, E., W. Bockting, M. Botzer, P. Cohen-Kettenis, G.
DeCuypere, J. Feldman, L. Fraser, et al. 2012. "Standards
of Care for the Health of Transsexual, Transgender, and
Gender-Nonconforming People." *International Journal of
Transgenderism* 13(4): 165–232. https://doi.org/10.1080
/15532739.2011.700873.

Crear-Perry, J., R. Correa-de-Araujo, T. L. Johnson, M. R.
McLemore, E. Neilson, and M. Wallace. 2020. "Social and
Structural Determinants of Health Inequities in Maternal
Health." *Journal of Women's Health*. https://doi.org/10.1089
/jwh.2020.8882.

Daniels, A. K. 1987. "Invisible Work." *Social Problems* 34(5) (December): 403–415.

Danielson, R., J. T. Wallenborn, D. K. Warne, and S. W. Masho. 2018. "Disparities in Risk Factors and Birth Outcomes among American Indians in North Dakota." *Maternal and Child Health Journal* 22: 1519–1525. https://doi.org/10.1007/s10995-018-2551-9.

Declercq, E. 2012. "Trends in Midwife-Attended Births in the United States, 1989–2009." *Journal of Midwifery and Women's Health* 57(4): 321–326. https://doi.org/10.1111/j.1542-2011.2012.00198.x.

Dekker, R. 2013. "Evidence Confirms Birth Centers Provide Top-Notch Care." Perkiomenville, PA: American Association of Birth Centers.

Gay and Lesbian Medical Association. 2006. *Guidelines for the Care of Lesbian, Gay, Bisexual, and Transgender Patients.* http://glma.org/_data/n_0001/resources/live/GLMA%20guidelines%202006%20FINAL.pdf.

Gonzalez, N. 2020. "Making the Case for Indigenous Midwifery: Battling White Saviors' Conquest for Control." Indigenous Goddess Gang. https://www.indigenousgoddessgang.com/home-1/2020/7/11/making-the-case-for-indigenous-midwifery-battling-white-saviors-conquest-for-control.

Grant, J. M., L. A. Mottet, and J. Tanis. 2011. "Injustice at Every Turn: A Report of the National Transgender Discrimination Survey." Washington, DC: National Center for Transgender Equality.

Gregory, K. D., S. Jackson, L. Korst, and M. Fridman. 2012. "Cesarean versus Vaginal Delivery: Whose Risks? Whose Benefits?" *American Journal of Perinatology* 29(1): 7–18.

Guise, J. M., K. Eden, C. Emeis, M. A. Denman, N. Marshall, R. R. Fu, R. Janik, et al. 2010. "Vaginal Birth after Cesarean:

New Insights." Washington, DC: Agency for Healthcare Research and Quality.

Health Management Associates. 2007. *Midwifery Licensure and Discipline Program in Washington State: Economic Costs and Benefits*. Olympia, WA: Washington State Dept. of Health, 1–31.

Hill, I., L. Dunbay, B. Courtot, S. Benatar, B. Garrett, F. Blavin, E. Howell, et al. 2014. *Strong Start for Mothers and Newborns Evaluation: Year 1 Annual Report*. Vol. 1, *Cross-Cutting Synthesis of Findings*. Washington, DC: Urban Institute.

Hinckley, D. 2014. "Average American Watches 5 Hours of TV per Day, Report Shows." *Daily News*, March 5.

Hochschild, A. R. 2012. *The Outsourced Self: Intimate Life in Market Times*. New York: Metropolitan Books.

Hoffkling, A., J. Obedin-Maliver, and J. Sevelius. 2017. "From Erasure to Opportunity: A Qualitative Study of the Experiences of Transgender Men around Pregnancy and Recommendations for Providers." *BMC Pregnancy and Childbirth* 17(2): 332.

Howell, E., A. Palmer, S. Benatar, and B. Garrett. 2014. "Potential Medicaid Cost Savings from Maternity Care Based at a Freestanding Birth Center." *Medicare and Medicaid Research Review* 4(3): E1–E13.

International Confederation of Midwives. 2017. "Human Rights of Lesbian, Gay, Bisexual, Transgender and Intersex (LGBTI) People." Strengthening Midwifery Globally. https://www.internationalmidwives.org/assets/files /statement-files/2018/04/eng-lgtbi.pdf.

Johantgen, M., L. Fountain, G. Zangaro, R. Newhouse, J. Stanic-Hutt, and K. White. 2012. "Comparison of Labor and Delivery Care Provided by Certified Nurse-Midwives and Physicians: A Systematic Review, 1990 to 2008." *Women's Health Issues* 22(1): e73–e81.

Jones, D. S. 2006. "The Persistence of American Indian Health Disparities." *American Journal of Public Health* 96(12): 2122–2134. https://doi.org/10.2105/AJPH.2004.054262.

Khazan, O. 2020. "The High Cost of Having a Baby in America." *The Atlantic*, January 6.

Klaus, M. H., J. H. Kennel, and P. H. Klaus. 2002. *The Doula Book: How a Trained Labor Companion Can Help You Have a Shorter, Easier and Healthier Birth*. Cambridge, MA: Perseus.

Kline, K. 2007. "Midwife Attended Births in Prime-Time Television: Craziness, Controlling Bitches and Ultimate Capitulation." *Women and Language* 30(1): 20–29.

Luce, A., M. Cash, V. Hundley, H. Cheyne, E. van Teijlingen, and C. Angell. 2016. "Is It Realistic? The Portrayal of Pregnancy and Childbirth in the Media." *BMC Pregnancy and Childbirth* 16: 40. https://doi.org/10.1186/s12884-016-0827-x.

Lutz, A. 2012. "These 6 Corporations Control 90% of the Media in America." Business Insider, June 14.

MacDonald, T., J. Noel-Weiss, D. West, M. Walks, M. L. Biener, A. Kibbe, and E. Myler. 2016. "Transmasculine Individual's Experiences with Lactation, Chest Feeding, and Gender Identity: A Qualitative Study." *BMC Pregnancy and Childbirth* 16: 106. https://doi.org/10.1186/s12884-016-0907-y.

Martin, J. A., B. E. Hamilton, M. J. K. Osterman, S. C. Curtin, and T. J. Matthews. 2015. "Births: Final Data for 2013." *National Vital Statistics Reports* 64(1): 1–65.

Martin, J. A., B. E. Hamilton, M. J. K. Osterman, A. K. Driscoll, and P. Drake. 2017. "Births: Final Data for 2017." *National Vital Statistics Reports* 67(8): 1–50.

Maura, C. 2019. "American College of Nurse-Midwives Issues Statement Strongly Opposing Withdrawal of Gender

Identity Protections in Health Care." Silver Spring, MD: American College of Nurse-Midwives.

Michal, C. A., P. A. Janssen, S. Vedam, E. K. Hutton, and A. de Jonge. 2011. "Planned Home vs. Hospital Birth: A Meta-Analysis Gone Wrong." *Medscape.* https://www.medscape.com/viewarticle/739987.

Midwives Alliance North America. 2014. "Use of Inclusive Language." https://mana.org/healthcare-policy/use-of-inclusive-language.

Moniz, M. H., A. Mark Fendrick, G. E. Kolenic, A. Tilea, L. K. Adman, and V. K. Dalton. 2020. "Out of Pocket Spending for Maternity Care among Women with Employer-Based Insurance, 2008–15." *Maternal and Child Health* 39(1): 18–23.

National Association of Certified Professional Midwives. 2014. "Commitments." https://nacpm.org/about-nacpm/about-the-organization/commitments/.

National Association to Advance Black Birth. 2018. "Black Birthing Bill of Rights." https://thenaabb.org/black-birthing-bill-of-rights/.

Novoa, C., and L. Truschel. 2018. "American Indian and Alaska Native Maternal and Infant Mortality: Challenges and Opportunities." Washington, DC: Center for American Progress.

Obedin-Maliver, J., and H. J. Makadon. 2015. "Transgender Men and Pregnancy." *Obstetric Medicine* 9(1): 4–8. https://doi.org/10.1177/1753495X15612658.

Raphael, D. 1973. *The Tender Gift: Breastfeeding.* Englewood Cliffs, NJ: Prentice-Hall.

Rayburn, W. F. 2011. *The Obstetrician-Gynecologist Workforce in the United States: Facts, Figures, and Implications, 2011.* Washington, DC: American Congress of Obstetricians and Gynecologists.

Ross, L. J., and R. Solinger. 2017. *Reproductive Justice: An Introduction*. Berkeley: University of California Press.

Schmidt, S. 2019. "A Mother, but Not a Woman." *Washington Post*. https://www.washingtonpost.com/.

Shah, N. 2015. "A NICE Delivery: The Cross-Atlantic Divide over Treatment Intensity in Childbirth." *New England Journal of Medicine* 372: 2181–2183.

SisterSong. n.d. "Reproducive Justice." Accessed January 21, 2021. https://www.sistersong.net/reproductive-justice.

Tribal Public and Environmental Health Think Tank. 2018. "Priorities in Tribal Public Health." Washington, DC: American Public Health Association.

Truven Health Analytics. 2013. *The Cost of Having a Baby in the United States*. Greenwood Village, CO: Truven.

Vitek, K., and M. Ward. 2019. "Risky, Dramatic, and Unrealistic: Reality Television Portrayals of Pregnancy and Childbirth and Their Effects on Women's Fear and Self-Efficacy." *Health Communication* 34(11): 1289–1295. https://doi.org/10.1080/10410236.2018.1481708.

Wax, J. R., F. L. Lucas, M. Lamont, M. G. Pinette, M. G. Cartin, and J. Blackstone. 2010. "Maternal and Newborn Outcomes in Planned Home Birth vs. Planned Hospital Births: A Metaanalysis." *American Journal of Obstetrics and Gynecology* 203(3): 243.E1–243.E8.

Wier, L. M., A. Pfuntner, J. Maeda, E. Stranges, K. Ryan, P. Jagadish, S. B. Collins, et al. 2011. "HCUP Facts and Figures: Statistics on Hospital-Based Care in the United States, 2009." Washington, DC: Agency for Healthcare Research and Quality.

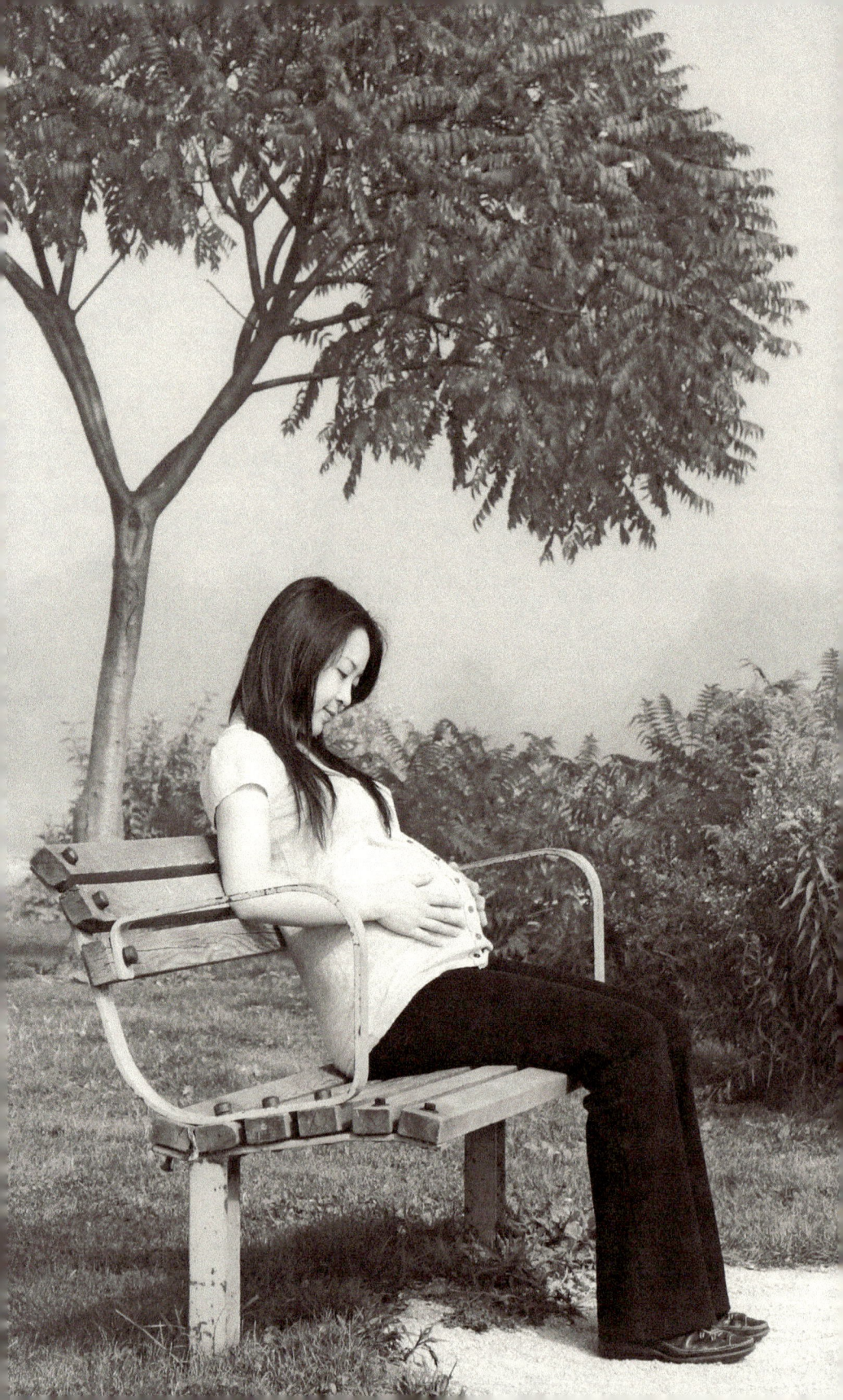

This chapter is an introduction to pregnancy and birth in the United States from the perspective of parents, providers, scholars, policy experts, and activists. The 10 essays in this chapter represent an exploration of topics not otherwise detailed in the book, but they are essential to understanding the complexities of pregnancy, birth, and parenthood in the United States.

Perinatal Loss
Meagan Lyon Leimena

Perinatal Loss: What Has Been Lost, and What Remains?

Perinatal loss is a profoundly difficult and complex experience for a woman and her family and has lasting psychological and social implications. And yet many of these losses are unseen, unacknowledged, or socially unrecognized, compounding the distress of women and their families. *Perinatal loss*, using a combination of definitions used in the United States and internationally, is the death of an infant less than 28 days of age or a fetus of less than 28 weeks gestation (Barfield 2016). *Early pregnancy loss*, with its complexities and grief trajectories (both explicit and ambiguous), is commonly defined as a loss before 20 weeks gestation (Barfield 2016). It could be related to infertility or a singular unexplained event and is quite common.

A pregnant person looking at their growing belly on a park bench. (Rgbe/Dreamstime.com)

These are powerful events in a woman's reproductive and family life.

Using a wide lens, perinatal death can represent interruption, transformation, or the end of a significant period of a woman's life, when she is making choices about having and raising children, sharing parenthood with a partner, and perhaps grappling with her own mortality and the extension of self that having a child, with the presumption that the child will outlive the parent, can have. The loss of a pregnancy or infant impacts a woman's sense of identity, both personal and social.

What Is Knowable about Perinatal Loss?

Perinatal loss is a prism through which to understand the intersection of tender human experience and the health care system. Women experiencing perinatal loss are vulnerable to health care providers, professionals, and systems that are poorly designed to understand and support the fullness of her losses. There is great variation in the language used for pregnancy loss, including, for example, *spontaneous abortion* and *products of conception*, which are often used in medical settings and can feel sanitized, uncomfortable, or misaligned with a woman's experience of her pregnancy. Similarly, *miscarriage* can feel vaguely punitive as a description, as though there was somehow fault or error on the part of the woman.

This gets to a larger, more obtuse issue about how knowable a woman's experience of pregnancy loss can be. As a deeply interior experience, perhaps known only to her or often played out in the less private spaces of hospitals, physicians' offices, and pharmacies, it may feel irreconcilable. Comparably, perinatal loss is a socially taboo subject, often spoken about in hushed tones, with whispered euphemisms, averted eyes, and an intolerance to process the fullness of loss, grief, and pain. Many wish to dismiss it entirely, downgrade its importance, or hurry along the processing of the loss (Lang 2011). A painful social convention is the notion that another pregnancy or infant will replace or remedy a loss, inadvertently negating the value of the lost pregnancy or infant.

Perinatal death is out of order, in whatever form it takes. "The universe breaks a sacred contract" (Inglis 2018). There is a death in the place where life begins, perhaps for some a more ambiguous ending even before a beginning, a hollowness where roundness belongs. An infant dying before her parents, without ever leaving a hospital room or opening her eyes, can be difficult to tolerate and honor. The death of a sibling anticipated and already loved who will never come home can feel impossible to explain and painful to integrate into a family narrative.

There is not only the loss of an infant, regardless of the developmental stage, but also the loss of a future and a life unlived, the transformation of a family by the legacy of absence. Consider the meaning of a significant date, such as a birthday for an elderly deceased family member. The annual anniversary of this date might bring a mix of sadness and fondness, of longing for more time but gratitude for the time shared, of memories and legacies built and celebrated over time. Now consider the meaning of the same significant date, a birthday, but for an infant who died the same day. This birthday, and date of death, represents not only the expanse of emotions about joining and leaving the world at once but also a life trajectory cut short. In lieu of memories, there is absence and space for what was not to be. This might include milestones unmet, experience never known, love unactualized, and a family altered.

There is appropriate sensitivity and caution around research with bereaved parents, but there are some themes that commonly emerge in literature about priorities for parents whose infants have died. Meaning making, or wanting to assign value to circumstances and events; recognizing the importance of the personhood they have assigned to their infant; and having opportunities to parent—in utero or after birth—and to make thoughtful choices for their child are a few of these (Nuzum,

Meeney, and O'Donoghue 2018). This can look like naming, bathing, and dressing their infant; having a detailed birth plan; having uninterrupted time as a family after delivery; and birth or death rituals that have cultural or religious value to the family.

There is great variation to the reactions, feelings, and needs of women after a perinatal loss. But it can be universally agreed that women deserve medical and psychosocial care that is attuned to their individuality, culturally humble, curious, and unhurried. For those who have lost what is most precious, the least we can offer is compassionate accompaniment and time as they traverse their grief.

A Challenge

[After all], grief serves a vital purpose in life. Grief is not an illness to cure or a disease to overcome. Mourning is an inherent aspect of wellness, as long as mortality defines our existence.

—Amy Wright Glenn (2017)

Are we able to look into this vast, painful human experience and hold space for the full complement of feelings and grief reactions? How can all health care providers encountering perinatal loss and those it touches be more attuned to their unique needs? Can we, socially and systemically, embrace the ideals of Reproductive Justice to hold space and honor the experiences of *all* women enduring perinatal loss, seeing in this call an opportunity to join more fully in the pursuit of equitable compassion and less othering? How can we amplify and better listen to the range of voices living through perinatal loss so that research, narratives, and the resultant policy decisions do not reflect hegemony and prize only voices who are privileged?

There is no single voice of perinatal loss, nor is there a singular path of grief. Kate Inglis, a mother who lost one of her twin babies and the author of *Notes for the Everlost: A Field Guide to Grief*, offers, "We integrate suffering by sharing it." Recognizing and holding space for the authentic and often painful experiences any woman knows after losing a pregnancy or infant is an important place we can collectively begin.

References

Barfield, W. D. 2016. "Standard Terminology for Fetal, Infant and Perinatal Deaths." *Pediatrics* 137(5). https://doi.org/10.1542/peds.2016-0551.

Glenn, A. W. 2017. *Holding Space: On Loving, Dying and Letting Go.* Berkeley, CA: Parallax Pres.

Inglis, K. 2018. *Notes for the Everlost: A Field Guide to Grief.* Boulder, CO: Shambhala.

Lang, A., A. R. Fleiszer, F. Duhamel, W. Sword, K. R. Gilbert, and S. Corsini-Munt. 2011. "Perinatal Loss and Parental Grief: The Challenge of Ambiguity and Disenfranchised Grief." *OMEGA—Journal of Death and Dying* 63(2): 183–196. https://journals.sagepub.com/doi/10.2190/OM.63.2.e.

Nuzum, D., S. Meeney, and K. O'Donoghue. 2018. "The Impact of Stillbirth on Bereaved Parents: A Qualitative Study." *PLOS One* 13(1). https://doi.org/10.1371/journal.pone.0191635.

Meagan Lyon Leimena has a BA in sociology from the University of Dayton, an MPH from the George Washington University, and an MSW from New York University. Ms. Leimena blends public health and social work in practice, writing, and teaching, with focus on perinatal health, pregnancy loss, and palliative care. Working as a consultant and coexecutive director of Babies Need Bottoms Diaper Bank, she is committed to the principles of social justice and dismantling oppressive structures.

Adoption
Barbara Katz Rothman

My own perspective on the issue of adoption is complex: I write as a feminist who has studied birth, called for the rights and power of women in childbirth, and argued for an understanding of pregnancy as a relationship and birth as an accomplishment of a woman's body. Babies are not, I have argued, "delivered" or "brought into the world." They do not come from hospitals. Babies grow in someone's body and are birthed by that person. And I write as a mother of two children by birth and one by adoption, a baby I "brought home" at eight days of age.

The very word *adoption* is problematic: one adopts pets, highways, textbooks, political platforms, and, yes, children. And plenty of people have objected to these other uses of the word, mostly claiming that it trivializes the concept. It feels wrong to use this same word for my relationship with my cat let alone my decision to use a particular textbook in a class I teach or some business's decision to sponsor highway cleanup campaigns. But what all the uses of the word, used in this broad way, imply is taking something foreign, an other, and making it one's own.

Adoption is taking a child and making that child one's own. And yet we also, in contemporary American discourse, routinely distinguish between a child "by adoption" and a child "of one's own." The fact of being adopted is forever in the present tense—I am an adoptive parent; she is an adopted child—and so the otherness, the foreignness of the child and the parent, are continually reinforced in our language. I have seen obituaries that report people as the "adopted" children of their parents.

What is it that makes that child "other"? Wherein lies the consistent, abiding foreignness of the adopted child to the adoptive family? It is certainly not how we feel; like every adoptive mother I have ever talked to, I feel no less the mother of my child by adoption than of my children by birth. Much has been written about this otherness from the side of the adoptees. They are the people living the Freudian family romance, the dream that there is, somewhere else, a better, truer, and more real set of parents, people who would really understand us. Like most dreams, it has its dark side. It has been common practice in the United States for records of adoption to be "sealed," with new birth certificates issued declaring the adoptive parents as the only parents. The first such sealed records were in Minnesota in 1917, but by the 1940s, most states had followed suit. Secrecy became built into adoption, with adoptees and birth parents having no access to any information let alone a relationship with each other.

In the 1970s, that began to shift as adoptees started to search for and find their birth parents. It was usually the birth mother that adoptees sought and were able to find. More states began to permit adult adoptees to have access to their original birth certificates. Coming out of the sealed records era, the drama of the search captured the imagination of the adoptee as well as the culture. Finding one's "real" family became expected. Medical histories were declared increasingly important, and the idea of genetic disease heritage legitimized the search.

It is also important to realize that over the course of that history, from the introduction of adoption as a legal concept at all to the situation we face now, adoption has changed from being a solution for children needing homes to a solution for people who want babies but are not able to produce their own. Adoption did not exist in English common law and was created by statute in Massachusetts in 1851, focused on protecting the "best interests" of the child. One of the concerns was to protect the child from the stigma of being a "bastard," a child born out of wedlock. Hiding the adoption, not only sealing the records but also trying to keep the adoption itself a secret, became socially valued. Women who became pregnant out of wedlock wanted to keep that secret and so were "sent away," with the pregnancy concealed. And adoptive parents sometimes concealed the fact of the adoption, faking a pregnancy or going away and returning as if they had birthed the child. The child was being protected.

Over time, adoption became less about finding homes for unplaced infants and more about meeting needs for babies. Because adoption solves, in a wonderful and satisfying way, the problem of infertility for so many people, we tend to forget that adoption itself is a problem and not just a solution. In countries that have good social services, readily available contraception as well as abortion, decent services for single mothers, guaranteed income, good publicly available education, parental leave, publicly funded medical insurance, and so on, it is quite rare for a pregnancy to end in adoption. It is in the poor countries, the countries without solid public infrastructure to protect families—and this sadly includes the United States along with many third world countries—that we find babies being made available for adoption. Rather than being about "child saving," as it used to be understood, following World War I, adoption in the United States was increasingly marketed to infertile couples as a way to meet their need for parenthood. And that is very much today's understanding of adoption: a beautiful way to form a family.

It is only inside of that perspective that the notion of a "baby shortage" makes any sense at all. If adoption was about helping parentless children, the absence of children in need would be a good thing. But adoption increasingly became a way to meet the needs of middle-class white people for the children they needed to complete their families. When the kinds of children they wanted were not available, they looked farther afield and began crossing borders, both class and racial borders within the country and foreign borders, developing a market for "international adoption."

I came to my own decision to adopt not out of infertility but at a moment in time when there were babies—Black babies—needing homes and not enough Black families with the wherewithal to adopt them. As a white family living in a Caribbean neighborhood in Brooklyn, we felt we could adopt such a child. I have addressed the complexities of being a white mother of a Black child in a book, Weaving a Family: Untangling Race and Adoption (Beacon Press, 2005).

The issue to be considered here, in a book focused on childbirth, is what are we to make of the relationship between the birth mother and the child she bears when she does not participate in raising that child? I draw upon the words of Ruth Hubbard, a biologist at Harvard University, who said that pregnancy "casts a shadow" over the first weeks of life, a period of early infancy in which the baby is missing its mother and the mother the baby in very clear physical ways. Babies have learned to recognize their birth mother's voice and language in pregnancy. The amniotic fluid in which they float in utero is scented with the mother's diet. When that same woman is nurturing that baby, there is a continuity that exists for both of them. With adoption, that continuity is lost. Even if the baby is held, loved, nurtured, and taken care of, there is an experience of strangeness. And the mother's body, even without the baby, will attempt to produce milk and continue into the postpartum period as a new mother.

Over time, the baby learns to turn to those who are nurturing him or her, to recognize their smell, their language, and their touch and to be soothed by those things. At a few months of age, the birth mother would be the foreign one and the adoptive family the safe comfort. While our language and cultural thinking act as if adoption were an ongoing state of affairs, the lived experience is that the adoption fades into the background, and the baby and parents bond, connect, and attach. The shadow of pregnancy fades.

Barbara Katz Rothman, PhD, is a professor of sociology, women's studies, and public health at the City University of New York, Baruch College and Graduate Center. She has been working on issues related to pregnancy and birth throughout her career.

Surrogacy
Renate Klein

Celebrities such as the Kardashians and Elton John and his husband are increasingly normalizing surrogacy. Can't make your own baby? Find yourself a "gestational carrier" to do it for you.

It is her "choice" to be a baby carrier and my "right" to have a baby that has part of my genes. When we see surrogacy discussed in the global media, it is in the form of feel-good stories about babies for couples that are desperate for their own child but are unable to have one naturally. What is not discussed is how, and more importantly by whom, the baby is made.

In the few countries where commercial surrogacy is legal (Ukraine, Georgia, Russia, Armenia, and 12 states in the United States), the woman who carries the baby is called the *gestational carrier, surrogate,* or *surrogate mother.* All these terms are entirely inappropriate, as there is nothing "surrogate" about this woman: she is the birth mother who grows the commissioned child from her own blood and bones.

In the United States, a so-called surrogate gets paid between $20,000 and $35,000, which amounts to less than $4 per hour. For the commissioning parents, the surrogacy can easily cost $100,000 or more because the birth mother often does not get pregnant or miscarries, so the procedure needs to be repeated more than once. Meanwhile, most of that money has turned the surrogacy industry into a billion-dollar enterprise: IVF clinics, brokers, lawyers, counselors, egg "donor" agencies, lobby groups, and other intermediaries. It is they who are exploiting this latest business opportunity to line their pockets.

In my book *Surrogacy: A Human Rights Violation,* I describe the surrogacy industry in greater detail (Klein 2017). I suggest that however great the pain caused by infertility, or however great the desire to have one's "own" genetic child, nothing in the world can justify putting the lives of two other human beings—the surrogate mother and the egg donor—at risk of short- and long-term physiological and psychological health problems that can be caused by IVF drugs and procedures as well as pregnancy and birth complications.

Surrogacy is a clear human rights violation. It is a practice of exploitation that violates a number of UN conventions and other international treaties. For instance, surrogacy can be likened to slavery, which Article 1 of the United Nations "Slavery

Convention" defines as "the status or condition of a person over whom any or all of the powers attaching to the right of ownership are exercised" (League of Nations 1926). When a woman agrees to be a surrogate, she surrenders control over her life for the next nine months. The commissioning parents (and their physician) decide what she eats and drinks, who she has sex with and how often, and how many tests she has to undergo to make sure the baby she carries has no "defects." If this "quality control" reveals imperfections, she can be forced to undergo an abortion; if more than one embryo was implanted and develops, fetal reduction can be mandated.

As the chair of the Scottish Council on Human Bioethics, Dr. Calum MacKellar, put it, "Selling surrogacy is a step towards slavery as women are dehumanized" (MacKellar 2019). And the director of Spain's Bioethics Committee, Federico de Montalvo, has made it clear that Spain will not be legalizing surrogacy, an unethical practice that "turns children into consumer objects" (de Montalvo 2019).

Surrogacy also profoundly violates the rights of the child. Under the United Nations *Convention on the Rights of the Child*, Article 2 prohibits the sale of children, and Article 35 stipulates that "State Parties shall take all appropriate national, bilateral and multilateral measures *to prevent the abduction of, the sale of, or traffic in children for any purpose or in any form*" (United Nations n.d.; emphasis added). In surrogacy, children are clearly sold.

Surrogacy also contravenes Article 1 of the "Optional Protocol to the *Convention on the Rights of the Child* on the Sale of Children, Child Prostitution and Child Pornography," which obligates governments to penalize the sale of children (United Nations 2002). Proponents of surrogacy say that the birth mother is paid for her "services," but this is blatantly untrue. If she miscarries or has an abortion, she will most likely not be paid. It is the "product child" that the payment is for.

In March 2017, the Italian feminist group Se Non Ora Quando—Libere ("If Not Now When—Free"), presented a request to the United Nations to address surrogacy in the *Convention of the Elimination of All Forms of Discrimination against Women* (CEDAW). The group asked the United Nations "to adopt—in the framework of CEDAW—a recommendation against surrogate motherhood on the model of the one adopted to fight female genital mutilation practices" because "surrogate motherhood leads to a real dehumanization of mother and child as it consciously creates a state of sacrifice and abandonment" (Se Non Ora Quando—Libere 2017). The United Nations has yet to respond.

Surrogacy supporters argue that women choose or consent to be surrogates, exercising their reproductive autonomy. Women are told to dissociate from the growing child on the basis that the embryo was made from the gametes of the commissioning parents (sperm from the male and the egg cell from his female partner or an unrelated egg donor—which is always the case when the commissioning parents are two men). Put differently, they claim that the fetus has nothing to do with the birth mother. Such pronouncements contradict the scientific knowledge that during pregnancy, cells are exchanged between mother and fetus and can remain in the woman's body decades after giving birth (Dawe, Tan, and Xiao 2007). Moreover, surrogacy proponents ignore the relationship that forms between a pregnant woman and her developing child—even when the mother's embryo/fetus was not made with her own egg cell—and how this might complicate the mother's attachment to the child and consequently her well-being after birth when she has her baby taken away. In surrogacy, most births end with a cesarean section (a C-section), putting the mother at greater risk and also more easily enabling the separation from the birth mother so that she often does not even see her child before he or she is taken away and delivered—like a product—to the people who paid for him or her.

In the anthology *Broken Bonds: Surrogate Mothers Speak Out* (Lahl, Reist, and Klein 2019), 15 women tell their stories of being left traumatized by their experiences as surrogate mothers in the United States, Australia, Canada, Russia, India, the United Kingdom, and Romania. In Australia, where only "altruistic" surrogacy is allowed, so-called surrogate mothers are not spared incredible pain and trauma. One such woman, Odette (a pseudonym), writes about profound betrayal, distress, and regret. She carried a baby for her physically infertile cousin out of love and compassion but was treated with unexpected cruelty during the entire pregnancy. After giving birth to the baby, Odette was denied the right to see or receive knowledge of the child. Three years later, she has still not seen the child—even in a photograph—and she struggles with her mental health, deep regret, and anger.

Thousands of individuals and international groups, such as Stop Surrogacy Now (www.stopsurrogacynow.com), the International Coalition for the Abolition of Surrogate Motherhood (ICAMS, originated in France), Stop Womb Rental (originated in Spain), Stoppt Leihmutterschaft (originated in Austria), and FINRRAGE (originated in Australia), strongly believe that surrogacy and egg donation can never be ethical or successfully regulated: laws will always offer loopholes, and the well-lawyered pro-surrogacy lobby will make sure the industry thrives regardless. What they seek is to abolish surrogacy globally. Countries that include India, Thailand, Nepal, and Cambodia have already banned the practice, and it has never been permitted in France, Switzerland, Spain, Austria, and Germany (Australia, Sweden, Belgium, and the United Kingdom only allow so-called altruistic surrogacy).

To achieve this aim, *we need to reduce demand.* We need to make it absolutely clear that *no one* has a right to *create* a child at the expense of two women, the surrogate and egg donor, who are harmed and exploited in the process. It does not matter whether they are straight, gay, in a couple, or single: a right to a child exists for no one. There are many other ways to have children in one's life. For instance, in the state of Victoria, in Australia, permanent care is one such avenue. It is different from adoption, as the children keep their own name, cultural identity, and contact with their birth families, if they so choose. Becoming a regular feature in the life of children of one's friends and families is another rewarding path. Such love is as profound and as real as having half your genes in a child whose gestation and birth is a violation of human rights that results in incredible trauma to surrogate mothers and egg donors.

References

Dawe, G. S., X. W. Tan, and Z.-C. Xiao. 2007. "Cell Migration from Baby to Mother." *Cell Adhesion and Migration* 1(1): 19–27. https://www.ncbi.nlm.nih.gov/pmc /articles/PMC2633676/.

de Montalvo, F. 2019. "Comité de Bioética, 'Hay que retirar por un tiempo la patria potestad a los padres que no quieran vacunar.'" El Mundo, January 22. https://www.elmundo.es /espana/2019/01/22/5c460f2dfc6c837e1a8b4750.html.

Klein, R. 2017. *Surrogacy. A Human Rights Violation.* Mission Beach, Australia: Spinifex Press; *Mietmutterschaft. Eine Menschenrechtsverletzung.* Hamburg, Germany: Marta Press. https://marta-press.com/cms /verlagsprogramm-sachbuch/renateklein-mietmutterschaft.

Lahl, J., M. T. Reist, and R. Klein, eds. 2019. *Broken Bonds. Surrogate Mothers Speak Out.* Mission Beach, Australia: Spinifex Press.

League of Nations. 1926. "No. 1414: Slavery Convention: Signed at Geneva, September 25, 1926." https://treaties.un .org/doc/Treaties/1926/09/19260925%2003-12%20AM /Ch_XVIII_3p.pdf.

MacKellar, C. 2019. "Selling Surrogacy Is a Step towards Slavery as Women Are Dehumanized." *The Scotsman,* January 24. https://www.scotsman.com/news/opinion /selling-surrogacy-is-a-step-towards-slavery-as-women-are -dehumanised-1-4861066.

Se Non Ora Quando—Libere. 2017. "United Nations Resolution against Surrogate Motherhood." March 23. http://www.stopsurrogacynow.com/wp-content/uploads /2017/04/OnuResolution_-Se-non-ora-quando-Libere -FIRME.pdf.

United Nations. 2002. "Optional Protocol to the *Convention on the Rights of the Child* on the Sale of Children, Child Prostitution and Child Pornography." UN Human Rights, Office of the High Commissioner for Human Rights. https://www.ohchr.org/en/professionalinterest/pages /opsccrc.aspx.

United Nations. n.d. *Convention on the Rights of the Child.* UN Human Rights, Office of the High Commissioner for Human Rights. Accessed January 21, 2021. https://www .ohchr.org/en/professionalinterest/pages/crc.aspx.

Dr. Renate Klein is a biologist and social scientist and is the coauthor/ coeditor of 15 books dealing with feminist theory and reproductive health matters. She was an associate professor in Women's Studies at Deakin University in Melbourne and has been a women's health activist since the 1980s. In 1985, she was a founder of Feminist International Network of Resistance to Reproductive and Genetic Engineering (FINRRAGE), and in 2015, she was an original signatory of the global campaign Stop Surrogacy Now. In 2019, Renate Klein was a cofounder of Abolish Surrogacy (Australia) (ABSA).

Disability and Pregnancy
April B. Coughlin

Introduction

People with disabilities have been viewed and positioned in society as a burden, incapable, nonsexual, and less than human, undeserving of equal rights or access (Davis 2017), and these stereotypes have been amplified by negative, stigmatizing, and inaccurate portrayals of disability in media (Dunn 2015; Haller 2010). As a result, women with disabilities, a historically forgotten and underserved population, often get lost in the conversations and research around pregnancy and birth. Factors that contribute to the less visible status of women with disabilities in society and the medical fields may include a lack of professional medical training in the area of women's health and disability as well as inaccessible offices, services, and medical procedures.

Disability in Society and the Medical Field: Attitudes, Education, and Treatment

While strides have been made in recent years to increase the inclusion of people with disabilities in schools, society, and the workforce, knowledge about disability and women's health and pregnancy remains an area that is largely misunderstood and lacking, particularly in the medical field. Women with disabilities have been historically positioned as recipients of care rather than as caregivers. Through depictions in media, women with disabilities are often not portrayed as confident, sexual, and desirable beings, but rather as passive, dependent, and vulnerable. As a result of these negative and inaccurate stereotypes, women with disabilities may not be viewed by society at large as capable of becoming pregnant, giving birth, and caring for a child (Iezzoni et al. 2015). These framings have a powerful and far-reaching influence on the experience of being a woman, pregnant, and disabled (Barnett et al. 2018; Iezzoni and Mitra 2017; Tefera et al. 2017).

Many of these perceptions about their inadequacy to care for a child come from within the families or friends of the women with disabilities themselves (Powell et al. 2017). Family members often express doubt in the physical or mental competence and ability of a parent with a disability through questions such as, "Who is going to help you care for the child?" "How will you lift or carry the baby?" "What if your medical condition gets in the way of your responsibilities as a parent?" or "How will you keep your baby safe in an emergency?"

Just as there is a lack of understanding about disabilities in the media, society, and even individual families, what is often found is varying degrees of disability knowledge in the medical field as well, specifically in regard to women's health, pregnancy, and birth. Part of this can be attributed to an insufficiency of relevant literature and updated research in this area (Samuel et al. 2007). This is a major contributing factor as to why women with disabilities receive less information about sexual and reproductive health than their able-bodied counterparts. Oftentimes, physicians and mental health providers are unaware of the issues and are therefore unprepared to provide education and resources to women with disabilities (Walsh-Gallagher et al. 2013).

Perhaps one of the least discussed issues in health care for women with disabilities is gynecological care. Research shows that women with disabilities, while more likely to be seen by specialists, are actually less likely to visit a gynecologist (Sonalkar et al. 2020). Although health care providers receive education and training in all areas of the population, many medical programs do not include adequate focus on the topic of disability. They may provide a cursory look at disability language and etiquette when interacting with individuals with disabilities, but there is typically no specific or in-depth focus on women with disabilities and most certainly not on disability, sexuality, pregnancy, and birth (Kendall et al. 2003; Walsh-Gallagher et al. 2013).

Physicians and other medical personnel are often not comfortable enough to initiate conversations about sexuality and pregnancy. Increased training of staff on issues of disability and sexuality and encouraging medical professionals to initiate these conversations with patients can be a positive step forward. In addition, increasing knowledge about disability and the lived experience among physicians and other health professionals, such as physical therapists, psychologists, nurses, midwives, doulas, personal care attendants, and home health aides, can lead to positive conversations and attitudes when interacting with clients with disabilities, particularly in discussions about health, sexuality, and pregnancy (Hall, Collins, and Ireland 2018; Höglund, Lindgren, and Larsson 2013; Ramamurthy 2012; Redshaw et al. 2013). When the topics of sexuality and pregnancy are not addressed or are automatically dismissed by medical professionals, women with disabilities may receive the hidden message that sexuality is not important or that pregnancy is not possible or recommended. This must change, and the conversation begins with the medical professionals themselves.

Access to Women's Health Care Facilities and Services for Individuals with Disabilities

Many women with disabilities report physicians' offices and services (specifically in women's health care) to be largely inaccessible (Malouf, Henderson, and Redshaw 2017; Mazurkiewicz, Stefaniak, and Dmoch-Gajzlerska 2018; Mitra et al. 2016; Prilleltensky 2003). Some examples include inaccessible entrances without ramps or automatic doors, nonadjustable exam tables, mammogram machines that are not accessible to women who use mobility devices or who cannot ambulate, inaccessible bathrooms they are required to use to provide urine samples during their visit, and a lack of ASL interpreters as well as inaccessible websites and medical forms that are not provided in alternate electronic formats. With all of these barriers, many women may just say, "Why bother?" and as a result, they may not be seen by a gynecologist, potentially missing out on early detection and developing otherwise preventable health problems.

For women with disabilities who decide to conceive or are pregnant, their prenatal and postnatal care may be determined by which health care facility provides accessibility, meaning there is a lack of true choice, which could ultimately lead to subpar health care for mother and baby. No woman should have to compromise the health of herself or her baby because of lack of access to a midwife or physicians' office, services, or testing.

Recommendations

For women with disabilities who are considering becoming pregnant or who have already conceived or given birth, there are many physical, social, and attitudinal barriers encountered along the way. Women with disabilities are constantly placed in the unfair and dehumanizing position of having to prove themselves as capable and competent human beings who are able to properly care for a child. Access to accessible medical services and physicians who have a comprehensive understanding of disability may be scarce and often requires exercising self-advocacy for the right to quality health care. The decision and ability to become pregnant, give birth, and care for a child may be called into question by family members and those in the medical field. Therefore, it is important to recognize and anticipate these obstacles before conceiving but also not allow them to deter women in their decision making and desire to become mothers.

Finding the right physicians, occupational and physical therapists, nurses, home health aides, midwives, and doulas with knowledge and experience working with individuals with disabilities is essential. These individuals should have a general interest in working with, learning from, and providing support through pregnancy and in postnatal care (McGarry, Kroese, and Cox 2016; Ramamurthy 2012). Although it is important to learn to advocate for oneself, it also helps to have health care providers who have a working knowledge and understanding of disability and the unique needs that may arise. It is crucial to have health care providers who can ensure full access to the most comprehensive and high-quality health care and testing possible.

What needs to be done is changing people's perceptions of disability and taking the time to listen to women's specific concerns about health and disability. It is about making offices, exam tables, information, services, and life-saving early detection accessible to women with disabilities. Through conducting more in-service training and education about the specific needs and concerns of women with disabilities, we can continue the dialogue around these issues and increase awareness and knowledge among medical professionals.

Those working in the medical field should not feel hesitant to talk to their female patients with disabilities about sexuality, body image, the importance of gynecological care, and the topic of pregnancy and birth. Instead, this should become part of the conversation in appointments. Many women with disabilities report a desire to have more education around these issues when visiting their physicians or other health care providers (Parker and Yau 2012; Smeltzer et al. 2016). By including conversations about sexuality and sexual health along with the other areas covered during medical appointments, women with disabilities will feel like it is acceptable to discuss concerns they may have and ultimately view pregnancy and childbirth as possible.

References

Barnett, B., L. Potvin, H. Brown, and V. Cobigo. 2018. "Women with Intellectual and Developmental Disabilities: Their Perceptions of Others' Attitudes toward Their Pregnancy." *Journal on Developmental Disabilities* 23(2) (May 1): 99.

Davis, L. 2017. *The Disability Studies Reader*. 5th ed. New York: Routledge.

Dunn, P. A. 2015. *Disabling Characters: Representations of Disability in Young Adult Literature*. New York: Peter Lang.

Hall, J., V. Hundley, B. Collins, and J. Ireland. 2018. "Dignity and Respect during Pregnancy and Childbirth: A Survey of the Experience of Disabled Women." *BMC*

Pregnancy and Childbirth 18(1) (August 13): 328–341. https://doi.org/10.1186/s12884-018-1950-7.

Haller, B. A. 2010. *Representing Disability in an Ableist World: Essays on Mass Media.* Louisville, KY: Advocado Press.

Höglund, B., P. Lindgren, and M. Larsson. 2013. "Midwives' Knowledge of, Attitudes Towards and Experiences of Caring for Women with Intellectual Disability during Pregnancy and Childbirth: A Cross-Sectional Study in Sweden." *Midwifery* 29(8) (August): 950–955.

Iezzoni, L. I., and M. Mitra. 2017. "Transcending the Counter-Normative: Sexual and Reproductive Health and Persons with Disability." *Disability and Health Journal* 10(3) (July): 369–370.

Iezzoni, L. I., A. J. Wint, S. C. Smeltzer, and J. L. Ecker. 2015. "'How Did That Happen?' Public Responses to Women with Mobility Disability during Pregnancy." *Disability and Health Journal* 8(3) (July): 380–387.

Kendall, M., S. Booth, P. Fronek, D. Miller, and T. Geraghty. 2003. "The Development of a Scale to Assess the Training Needs of Professionals in Providing Sexuality Rehabilitation Following Spinal Cord Injury." *Sex Disability* 21: 49–64.

Malouf, R., J. Henderson, and M. Redshaw. 2017. "Access and Quality of Maternity Care for Disabled Women during Pregnancy, Birth and the Postnatal Period in England: Data from a National Survey." *BMJ Open* 7(7) (January 1): e016757.

Mazurkiewicz, B., M. Stefaniak, and E. Dmoch-Gajzlerska. 2018. "Perinatal Care Needs and Expectations of Women with Low Vision or Total Blindness in Warsaw, Poland." *Disability and Health Journal* 11(4) (October 1): 618–623.

McGarry, A., B. S. Kroese, and R. Cox. 2016. "How Do Women with an Intellectual Disability Experience the Support of a Doula during Their Pregnancy, Childbirth and after the Birth of Their Child?" *Journal of Applied Research in Intellectual Disabilities* 29(1) (January1): 21–33.

Mitra, M., L. M. Long-Bellil, L. I. Iezzoni, S. C. Smeltzer, and L. D. Smith. 2016. "Pregnancy among Women with Physical Disabilities: Unmet Needs and Recommendations on Navigating Pregnancy." *Disability and Health Journal* 9(3) (July): 457–463.

Parker, M., and M. Yau. 2012. "Sexuality, Identity and Women with Spinal Cord Injury." *Sex Disability* 30: 15–27.

Powell, R. M., M. Mitra, S. C. Smeltzer, L. M. Long-Bellil, L. D. Smith, and L. I. Iezzoni. 2017. "Family Attitudes and Reactions toward Pregnancy among Women with Physical Disabilities." *Women's Health Issues* 27(3) (May): 345–350.

Prilleltensky, O. 2003. "A Ramp to Motherhood: The Experiences of Mothers with Physical Disabilities." *Sexuality and Disability* 21(1) (March): 21–47.

Ramamurthy, K. 2012. "Meeting the Health Needs of Disabled Parents." *Community Practitioner* 85(3) (March 1): 34, 36.

Redshaw, M., R. Malouf, H. Gao, and R. Gray. 2013. "Women with Disability: The Experience of Maternity Care during Pregnancy, Labour and Birth and the Postnatal Period." *BMC Pregnancy and Childbirth* 13(1) (September 13): 14 pages.

Samuel, V. M., J. Moses, N. North, H. Smith, and K. Thorne. 2007. "Spinal Cord Injury Rehabilitation: The Experience of Women." *Spinal Cord* 45: 758–764.

Smeltzer, S. C., M. Mitra, L. I. Iezzoni, L. Long-Bellil, and L. D. Smith. 2016. "Perinatal Experiences of Women with Physical Disabilities and Their Recommendations for Clinicians." *Journal of Obstetric, Gynecologic & Neonatal Nursing* 45(6) (November): 781–789.

Sonalkar, S., V. Chavez, J. McClusky, T. A. Hunter, and C. J. Mollen. 2020. "Gynecologic Care for Women with

Physical Disabilities: A Qualitative Study of Patients and Providers." *Women's Health Issues* 30(2) (March): 136–141.

Tefera, B., M. Van Engen, J. Van Der Klink, and A. Schippers. 2017. "The Grace of Motherhood: Disabled Women Contending with Societal Denial of Intimacy, Pregnancy, and Motherhood in Ethiopia." *Disability & Society* 32(10) (November 26): 1510–1533.

Walsh-Gallagher, D., R. Mc Conkey, M. Sinclair, and R. Clarke. 2013. "Normalising Birth for Women with a Disability: The Challenges Facing Practitioners." *Midwifery* 29(4) (April 1): 294–299.

April B. Coughlin is a professor at the State University of New York at New Paltz in the School of Education. She also worked as a high school English teacher in New York City public schools. Her research focuses on access and equity for students with disabilities in schools and health care for women with disabilities. A "wheeler" since the age of six and a lifelong disability rights advocate, April is committed to increasing awareness and education about the need for physical access and inclusion for individuals with disabilities in schools and the community.

Empathy, Pregnancy, and Mental Health
Jozette Belmont

Pregnant people experience an array of stressors, including changes to their body, hormones, and everyday life. Yet, pregnant people who suffer from mental disabilities during and after pregnancy are rarely acknowledged. Approximately 15–29 percent of pregnant people are diagnosed with a mental disability, and it is likely that number would rise if more people felt comfortable seeking help (Moore and Pytlarz 2013, 83–87). For those who experience postpartum depression and psychosis, pregnancy and birthing can result in increased stress, suicidal thoughts, or hallucinations, which may not be properly cared for due to shame. Without access to care and support, pregnant people with mental disabilities have increased health risks and higher chances of suicidal thoughts, and they may be unable to care for themselves or their children (World Health Organization (WHO) 2015). It is critical that we approach pregnant people with mental disabilities with empathy and acknowledge the societal and physical stress pregnancy has on the body and mind.

On Language: Mental Disabilities and Pregnant People

It is important to note why I use the term "mental disabilities" over more common labels. In *Keywords for Disability Studies,* Rachel Adams, Benjamin Reiss, and David Serlin assert, "In the 'social model [of disability],' one is disabled because of the body's interaction with the social and physical environment rather than because of individual pathology or 'lack'" (Adams, Reiss, and Serlin 2015). To this effect, rather than define someone as *disordered* or *ill,* the term *mental disabilities* references the ways one's body and mind interacts with a world designed for nondisabled people. Additionally, wherever possible, I use the term *pregnant people* instead of *pregnant women,* as this is inclusive of all gender identities. Although most research and statistics only include self-identified women, this highlights the gap in current scholarship and the need for more inclusive practices.

Mental Health and Pregnancy: An Overview

According to Dr. Katherine J. Gold and Dr. Sheila M. Marcus, "Nearly half of Americans will have a mental illness in their lifetime. . . . Since the majority of these illnesses start before or during the child-bearing years, many pregnant women have significant psychiatric comorbidity" (Gold and Marcus 2008). *Comorbidity* is defined as two or more disorders occurring at the same time ("Comorbid" n.d.). In this case, pregnant people may experience two or more mental disabilities at once during a time when they are already undergoing increased stress and change. Statistics on pregnant people show 13.3 percent have a mood disorder, 13 percent have an anxiety disorder, and 0.4 percent have a psychotic disorder, and many cannot take medication that might help them (Effective Health Care Program 2019). This can be compounded by postpartum depression or psychosis, which may go unnoticed by support systems. Further, pregnant people may feel shame in expressing these emotions, especially given the societal expectations of new parents (WHO 2015). This is why we must validate pregnant people who have mental disabilities—so they feel comfortable seeking help.

Postpartum Depression and Psychosis

Postpartum depression (PPD) is defined as a period of at least two weeks where a pregnant person experiences depression, sleep disturbance, appetite changes, loss of energy, feelings of worthlessness or guilt, or suicidal thoughts. The onset of symptoms may start as early as the fifth month of pregnancy, but most experience it one month after giving birth (Pearlstein et al. 2009). According to the CDC, 11 percent of pregnant women experience PPD (Centers for Disease Control and Prevention 2020). In recent years, PPD has been widely discussed, although guilt and shame still occur. To combat this, efforts have been made to normalize discussions of PPD and warning signs are more accessible to support systems. Yet, the Mayo Clinic highlights the following risk factors of developing PPD: history of depression or bipolar disorder, personal history of PPD, family history of depression or PPD, experiencing a stressful event in the past year, or a strained relationship with one's support system (Mayo Clinic 2018). It is clear that pregnant people with a personal or familial history of mental disabilities should be identified and treated as soon as possible. However, it is also important to acknowledge that access to this requires adequate health care and good financial standing, which some may not have. Although PPD is more frequently discussed and addressed, there are still significant disparities for pregnant people and their support systems.

Consequently, postpartum psychosis (PPP) is often forgotten when addressing pregnant people's needs. PPP is defined as a period of at least two weeks following pregnancy where one may experience delusions, hallucinations, increased irritation, hyperactivity, decreased need or inability to sleep, paranoia, rapid mood swings, or difficulty communicating. Compared to PPD, PPP impacts pregnant people 1–2 percent of the time (Postpartum Support International (PSI) n.d.). However, diagnosis can be difficult, and the impacts of PPP are even more life threatening. Research suggests it has a 5 percent suicide completion rate and a 4 percent infanticide rate (PSI n.d.). Due to the increased risks to both the pregnant person and child, discussion of PPP tends to villainize the pregnant person instead of empathizing with them.

One example of the risks and stigma of PPP comes from the Andrea Yates case. Yates is known for killing her five children in 2001, which occurred during a period of PPP. Andrea and Russell Yates had their children in quick succession and did not use birth control due to religious beliefs. Yates had a history of experiencing hallucinations, and for at least two years, she had fantasized about killing her children to save them from her own perceived "bad motherhood." Yates had previously taken Haldol, an antipsychotic medication, to help her hallucinations and paranoia, but she had to stop taking it every time she got pregnant. In addition, her living situation with Russell was chaotic; at one point, the entire family lived in a small camping trailer. Many, including a jury who found her guilty of capital murder, felt she was fully to blame for the unfortunate deaths of her children. While these deaths are incomprehensible, the public scrutiny of Yates failed to acknowledge the social and psychological stressors she experienced (McLellan 2006; CNN editorial staff 2019).

Although difficult, if we were to take into account Andrea Yates's experiences, we would see a person who was not given adequate mental health care. While her familial religious beliefs should be upheld, Yates was also medically unwell.

Her mental health should have been centered so she could feel stable and supported. Cases like this should be identified and explored more deeply to inform parents of warning signs and risks. Prevention and treatment are pivotal to supporting pregnant people who experience PPD, PPP, and other mental disabilities.

Leading with Empathy

It is evident that pregnant people with mental disabilities may not receive adequate care. It is important to inform both the pregnant person and their support system of warning signs and what to do if something is wrong. It is up to medical professionals and the general public to destigmatize mental disabilities.

So, how can we make changes? First, medical professionals should uphold the importance of mental health as well as physical. A person's physical and mental well-being are deeply intertwined, and the safety of the pregnant person and fetus relies on their being treated with compassion and care. To address this, however, health care providers also need to widen their scope and more adequately address the needs of low-income pregnant people who may not have access to care (Garfield et al. 2015). Pregnant people and their support systems need access to warning signs, resources, and more avenues of support. Finally, *all of us* should acknowledge the prevalence of mental disabilities in pregnant people and find ways to support those who need it most. Judgment and stigma help no one get better. Even when things seem grim, we must recognize that everyone is coming from a different place, and we need to meet them there. Empathy and compassion should be at the heart of caring for every pregnant person.

References

Adams, R., B. Reiss, and D. Serlin. 2015. *Keywords for Disability Studies*. New York: New York University Press.

Centers for Disease Control and Prevention. 2020. "Depression among Women." April 8. https://www.cdc.gov /reproductivehealth/depression/index.htm.

CNN editorial staff. 2019. "Andrea Yates Fast Facts." CNN, June 14. https://www.cnn.com/2013/03/25/us /andrea-yates-fast-facts/index.html.

"Comorbid." n.d. *Merriam-Webster.com Dictionary*. Accessed April 12, 2020. https://www.merriam-webster.com /dictionary/comorbid#medicalDictionary.

Effective Health Care Program. 2019. "Maternal and Fetal Effects of Mental Health Treatments in Pregnant and Breastfeeding Women: A Systematic Review of Pharmacological Interventions." January 11. https:// effectivehealthcare.ahrq.gov/products/mental-health -pregnancy/protocol.

Garfield, L., D. Holditch-Davis, C. Sue Carter, B. L. McFarlin, D. Schwertz, J. S. Seng, C. Giurgescu, et al. 2015. "Risk Factors for Postpartum Depressive Symptoms in Low-Income Women with Very Low-Birth-Weight Infants." *Advances in Neonatal Care* 15(1): E3–E8. https:// doi.org/10.1097/anc.0000000000000131.

Gold, K. J., and S. M. Marcus. 2008. "Effect of Maternal Mental Illness on Pregnancy Outcomes." *Expert Reviews of Obstetrics & Gynecology* 3(3): 391–401. https://www .medscape.com/viewarticle/573947.

Mayo Clinic. 2018. "Postpartum Depression." Mayo Foundation for Medical Education and Research, September 1. https://www.mayoclinic.org/diseases-conditions /postpartum-depression/symptoms-causes/syc-20376617.

McLellan, F. 2006. "Mental Health and Justice: The Case of Andrea Yates." *The Lancet* 368(9551): 1951–1954. https:// doi.org/10.1016/s0140-6736(06)69789-4.

Moore, T., and J. Pytlarz. 2013. "Untreated Psychiatric Disorder in Pregnancy: Weighing the Risks." *Mental Health*

Clinician 3(2): 83–87. https://doi.org/10.9740/mhc.n163635.

Pearlstein, T., M. Howard, A. Salisbury, and C. Zlotnick. 2009. "Postpartum Depression." *American Journal of Obstetrics and Gynecology* 200(4): 357–364. https://www.ncbi.nlm.nih.gov/pmc/articles/PMC3918890/.

Postpartum Support International (PSI). n.d. "Postpartum Psychosis." Accessed April 13, 2020. https://www.postpartum.net/learn-more/postpartum-psychosis/.

World Health Organization (WHO). 2015. "Maternal Mental Health." February 20. https://www.who.int/mental_health/maternal-child/maternal_mental_health/en/.

Jozette Belmont (she/they) is a second year in the Women's and Gender Studies MA program at the Graduate Center, CUNY. Their research focuses on how sex education impacts queer people in New York State. They also work at Peer Health Exchange, a health education nonprofit, as a development and systems associate doing grant writing, fundraising, and data management. They hope to continue their work by contributing to ongoing scholarship and advocating for concrete systemic changes.

Intimate Partner Violence during Pregnancy: Health Consequences and Social Causes
Jennifer Leigh

Intimate partner violence (IPV) is an extremely prevalent form of gender-based violence; globally, about one in three women report experiencing IPV at some point during their lives (Black et al. 2010). Although a wide variety of behaviors can be understood as intimate partner violence, the Centers for Disease Control and Prevention (CDC) defines five types of IPV, including physical violence, sexual violence, psychological aggression, stalking, and control of reproductive/sexual health. As pregnancy is a time of increased need for physical, social, and financial support, it is also a time of greater vulnerability to violence. Most discourse around IPV during pregnancy focuses on the experiences of heterosexual cisgender women, as they comprise the majority of both pregnancies and cases of IPV; however, to reflect the experiences of all genders during pregnancy, the term *pregnant people* will be used throughout this piece.

Between 1 percent and 28 percent of pregnant people worldwide experience IPV (García-Moreno et al. 2005), with most surveys estimating a prevalence between 3.9 percent and 8.7 percent (Devries et al. 2010). This is potentially a higher prevalence than many health conditions that are routinely screened for as part of prenatal care, such as diabetes or preeclampsia. The risk of IPV during pregnancy is not experienced equally; people who are young, unmarried, racial and ethnic minorities, or of lower income and education levels have been consistently shown to be at greater risk (Janssen et al. 2003; Bohn, Tebben, and Campbell 2004).

Existing research has identified two patterns of violence against pregnant people. For individuals who had not previously experienced violence, pregnancy is a period when vulnerability to violence can be increased. For individuals who had already experienced violence, violence that continues through pregnancy can pose additional concerns for health and safety. Pregnant people are at risk for new manifestations of IPV throughout pregnancy, including forcing an unwanted pregnancy, refusing to pay for child-related expenses, cutting off access to prenatal care, and threatening to harm the fetus or child. Several studies have identified homicide as the leading cause of death for pregnant people, with a greater risk for young African American women (Cheng and Horon 2010).

Reproductive Coercion and Control

Intimate partner violence during pregnancy is often intertwined with reproductive coercion. Examples of reproductive coercion include refusing to use or tampering with birth control (e.g., poking holes in condoms), forced abortion, or forced continuation of pregnancy. This form of coercion can be exercised by either partner in a relationship. Importantly, reproductive coercion generally centers less on the pregnancy outcome; rather, it is about one partner maintaining a sense of power and control over the other.

Research on the association between reproductive coercion and IPV has been limited, with most studies emerging within the past decade. A national survey conducted by the National Domestic Violence Hotline in 2011 found that out of 3,000 calls to the hotline, 25 percent reported some form of reproductive coercion (National Domestic Violence Hotline 2011). Other studies have supported the link between reproductive coercion and other IPV behaviors, with one study reporting that three-quarters of individuals who reported pregnancy coercion or birth control sabotage also reported a history of other forms of IPV (Miller et al. 2010). Racial health disparities are reflected in reproductive coercion, with studies showing that 37.1 percent of Black and 29.0 percent of multiracial women reported reproductive coercion (Holliday et al. 2017). Despite the high prevalence of reproductive coercion, much remains unknown. Notably, as the majority of studies on reproductive coercion are cross-sectional, it is difficult to identify the temporal relationship between reproductive coercion and IPV (Grace and Anderson 2018).

Health Impacts of IPV during Pregnancy

Intimate partner violence during pregnancy is associated with substantial negative health outcomes for both the pregnant person and the child. People experiencing IPV may be less likely to attend their prenatal visits and receive continuous prenatal care (Dunn and Oths 2004). Experiencing physical violence during pregnancy puts pregnant people at an increased risk of antepartum hemorrhage and intrauterine growth restriction (Janssen et al. 2003). There are also notable consequences for the child's short- and long-term health; studies have also found that IPV during pregnancy is associated with increased risk of preterm birth and low infant birth weight (Shah and Shah 2010; Campbell 2002). Among the most severe impacts, experiences of IPV during pregnancy are associated with an increased risk of perinatal and neonatal death. In cases where the pregnant person gives birth after being hospitalized for a physical assault, studies found an eighteenfold increased risk of maternal death and a sevenfold increased risk of fetal death (El Kady, Smith, and Gilbert 2005). As in many studies related to the impacts of violence, the causal mechanisms of these effects remain unclear; however, available data show that IPV during pregnancy is a major and potentially lethal health concern.

Beyond the Medical Sphere: Addressing the Root Causes of Intimate Partner Violence

Intimate partner violence threatens not only the health and well-being of survivors but also their bodily autonomy and other freedoms that are all the more critical for pregnant people. As pregnant people generally receive ongoing medical care, health professionals are in a unique position to support pregnant survivors. To improve the identification of IPV during pregnancy and treatment for pregnant patients who have experienced violence, all health professionals should be trained in trauma-informed care. Ideally, mental health and social services can be integrated into patient care to connect patients who have experienced IPV to ongoing care and support. One such model is the EMPOWER Clinic in New York City, which offers colocated and collaborative obstetric-gynecological and psychiatric care (Ades et al. 2019).

However, attention paid to violence prevention should not stray from the social roots of violence. As IPV is often considered a private issue to be resolved between individuals, current approaches have treated it as separate from other forms of violence and oppression. In actuality, IPV is a manifestation of greater societal power inequities, namely sexism, racism, and classism, among others. The work of INCITE! Women of

Color against Violence centers these "dangerous intersections," incorporating IPV into a broader theory of transformative justice that connects sexual and gender-based violence with forms of institutionalized violence, such as militarism, mass incarceration, and colonialism (INCITE! Women of Color Against Violence n.d.). This perspective recognizes that the medical, criminal, and social welfare systems that often support survivors of IPV have in fact been a source of violence for many marginalized communities. For example, police are often first responders for people who are experiencing IPV, but these law enforcement–based approaches can be counterproductive and dangerous for survivors of color.

An emphasis on community-driven responses is critical to prioritize not only short-term survival but long-term healing. An increased focus on community care and organizing efforts that address the root causes of violence is critical in preventing the occurrence of violence and promoting Reproductive Justice.

References

Ades, V., S. X. Wu, E. Rabinowitz, S. Chemouni Bach, B. Goddard, S. P. Ayala, and J. Greene. 2019. "An Integrated, Trauma-Informed Care Model for Female Survivors of Sexual Violence: The Engage, Motivate, Protect, Organize, Self-Worth, Educate, Respect (EMPOWER) Clinic." *Obstetrics and Gynecology* 133(4): 803–809.

Black, M. C., K. C. Basile, M. J. Breiding, S. G. Smith, M. L. Walters, M. T. Merrick, J. Chen, et al. 2010. *The National Intimate Partner and Sexual Violence Survey: 2010 Summary Report*. Atlanta, GA: National Center for Injury Prevention and Control, Centers for Disease Control and Prevention.

Bohn, D. K., J. G. Tebben, and J. C. Campbell. 2004. "Influences of Income, Education, Age, and Ethnicity on Physical Abuse before and during Pregnancy." *Journal of Obstetric, Gynecologic, and Neonatal Nursing* 33(5): 561–571.

Campbell, J. C. 2002. "Health Consequences of Intimate Partner Violence." *The Lancet* 359(9314): 1331–1336.

Cheng, D., and I. L. Horon. 2010. "Intimate-Partner Homicide among Pregnant and Postpartum Women." *Obstetrics and Gynecology* 115(6): 1181–1186.

Devries, K. M., S. Kishor, H. Johnson, H. Stöckl, L. J. Bacchus, C. Garcia-Moreno, and C. Watts. 2010. "Intimate Partner Violence during Pregnancy: Analysis of Prevalence Data from 19 Countries." *Reproductive Health Matters* 18(36): 158–170.

Dunn, L. L., and K. S. Oths. 2004. "Prenatal Predictors of Intimate Partner Abuse." *Journal of Obstetric, Gynecologic, and Neonatal Nursing* 33(1): 54–63.

El Kady, D., L. Smith, and W. M. Gilbert. 2003. "Maternal and Neonatal Outcomes of Assaults and Intentional Injuries in Pregnancy." *American Journal of Obstetrics and Gynecology* 189(6): S120.

García-Moreno, C., H. Jansen, M. Ellsberg, L. Heise, and C. Watts. 2005. *WHO Multi-Country Study on Women's Health and Domestic Violence against Women: Initial Results on Prevalence, Health Outcomes and Women's Responses.* Geneva, Switzerland: World Health Organization.

Grace, K. T., and J. C. Anderson. 2018. "Reproductive Coercion: A Systematic Review." *Trauma, Violence, and Abuse* 19(4): 371–390.

Holliday, C. N., H. L. McCauley, J. G. Silverman, E. Ricci, M. R. Decker, D. J. Tancredi, J. G. Burke, et al. 2017. "Racial/Ethnic Differences in Women's Experiences of Reproductive Coercion, Intimate Partner Violence, and Unintended Pregnancy." *Journal of Women's Health* 26(8): 828–835.

INCITE! Women of Color against Violence. n.d. "INCITE!—Critical Resistance Statement." Accessed April 20, 2020. https://incite-national.org/incite-critical-resistance-statement/.

Janssen, P. A., V. L. Holt, N. K. Sugg, I. Emanuel, C. M. Critchlow, and A. D. Henderson. 2003. "Intimate Partner Violence and Adverse Pregnancy Outcomes: A Population-Based Study." *American Journal of Obstetrics and Gynecology* 188(5): 1341–1347.

Miller, E., M. R. Decker, H. L. McCauley, D. J. Tancredi, R. R. Levenson, J. Waldman, P. Schoenwald, et al. 2010. "Pregnancy Coercion, Intimate Partner Violence, and Unintended Pregnancy." *Contraception* 81: 316–322.

National Domestic Violence Hotline. 2011. "1 in 4 Callers to the National Domestic Violence Hotline Report Birth Control Sabotage and Pregnancy Coercion." https://www.thehotline.org/news/1-in-4-callers-to-the-national-domestic-violence-hotline-report-birth-control-sabotage-and-pregnancy-coercion/.

Shah, P. S., and J. Shah. 2010. "Maternal Exposure to Domestic Violence and Pregnancy and Birth Outcomes: A Systematic Review and Meta-Analyses." *Violence Against Women* 19(11): 2017–2031.

Jennifer Leigh is a PhD student in the Department of Sociology at New York University. Her research focuses on the medicalization of violence and trauma as well as issues confronting the health care labor force. She received her BA in neuroscience and behavior and ethnomusicology from Barnard College and her MPH in socio-medical sciences from the Mailman School of Public Health.

Certified Professional Midwives: Leveraging Policy to Improve Health
Mary Lawlor

Certified professional midwives (CPMs) have a critical role to play in improving the health—and even saving the lives—of people giving birth in the United States today. In my two decades with the National Association of Certified Professional

Midwives (NACPM), I have learned about the plight of birthing people in our country, causing me to become a passionate advocate for midwives, for improving care for all birthing people, and for eliminating unconscionable racial inequities. It has been an exciting journey of learning about how NACPM can lead in leveraging policy for the benefit of birthing people and their babies.

Birth in the United States—A Risky Business

Giving birth in the United States can be a risky proposition. As a result of the hospitalization and medicalization of birth over the past century, we overuse expensive technologies and interventions, best reserved for sick people, to care for healthy pregnant people. Cesarean section, the most commonly performed surgery in the United States increased by 60 percent from 1996 to 2009. Although not associated with increased benefit, approximately one-third of all births in our country are by cesarean section.

In addition, we underuse many beneficial forms of care shown to protect and enhance the health of birthing people, including midwife care, continuous support during labor, and drug-free measures for comfort and progress in labor. In the United States, midwives attend 11 percent of births, while in Western European countries, where outcomes are better, midwives attend 60–80 percent of all births.

This overuse of interventions and underuse of beneficial forms of care has resulted in the most expensive perinatal system in the world along with mortality rates that are far worse than all other wealthy nations and even worse than many poorer nations. In 2014, 36 countries had a lower infant mortality rate, 62 had a lower rate of maternal death, and 97 had a higher rate of breastfeeding at 6 months than the United States The United States has the highest maternal death rate among developed countries and is the *only* wealthy nation where maternal mortality is rising.

Against this backdrop, the pregnancy and birth outcomes for people of color are shockingly worse than for white people.

Black people, regardless of social status, are 4 times more likely to die of pregnancy-related complications than their white counterparts, and their babies are 2.5 times more likely to die in their first year of life. American Indians and Alaska Natives have an infant death rate 60 percent higher than the rate for whites. Although these disparities may be due in part to unequal access to care, systemic racism has been shown to be a root cause.

What's a Midwife to Do?

In the United States, CPMs provide unique and critical access to normal physiologic birth (ACNM, MANA, and NACPM 2013) profoundly benefiting childbearing people and their babies. Although qualified to practice in any setting, CPMs have particular expertise in care in community settings, and they own or work in over half of the 350 birth centers in the United States. In these settings, away from the typical medical interventions experienced by most people giving birth today, CPMs have become experts in facilitating the innate processes of birth (National Association of Certified Professional Midwives (NACPM) 2017).

Time and again, research has demonstrated that the care of midwives enhances health and improves outcomes (*The Lancet* 2014). CPM care results in significantly fewer cesarean sections, low birth weight and premature babies, and much higher rates of breastfeeding than for healthy people in hospital care (Cheyney et al. 2014). In 2017, the Visionary Vanguard Group found that a CPM-led model in Florida eliminated health disparities in preterm birth outcomes and reduced low birth weight babies in at-risk populations (Visionary Vanguard Group 2017). A national report published by the Milbank Memorial Fund on Evidence-Based Maternity Care states that "the low CPM study rates of interventions are benchmarks for what the majority of childbearing women and babies who are in good health might achieve" (Sakala and Corry 2008). Reports out of Washington State indicate substantial cost savings with CPMs, especially as a result of cesarean section reduction (Health Management Associates 2007; Washington State Health Care Authority 2016). CPMs have an important role to play in leading efforts to improve outcomes for the birthing population and in eliminating racial inequities and disparities.

What's a Professional Association to Do?: CPMs and Health Policy

There is a critical and urgent need to make the benefits of CPM care available to all families, regardless of means, in every community. NACPM is committed to state and federal policy initiatives to secure a place a place for the unique and valuable services of CPMs and to driving urgently needed structural changes in the systems of care for birthing people in the United States today.

In the United States, defining and implementing health policy happens on both the state and federal levels. States have jurisdiction over licensing and regulation, while Medicaid, for example, is a state and federal partnership. Congress passes laws, such as the 2010 Affordable Care Act, that shape the way both federal and state governments deliver health care. Numerous federal agencies, such as the Centers for Medicare and Medicaid Services (CMS), interpret, implement, and enforce those laws. NACPM must engage on all these levels of policy.

State and Jurisdiction Policy

NACPM is committed to ensuring licensing for CPMs in all jurisdictions, a mechanism for protecting public health and safety and strengthening the role of the profession in defining safe, competent care. Licensure is a cornerstone for consumer access to health professions.

NACPM led in a several-year midwifery national collaboration—the United States Midwifery Education, Regulation, and Association (US MERA) (US Midwifery Education, Regulation, and Association (US MERA) n.d.)—that established Principles for Model U.S. Midwifery Legislation and Regulation (US MERA 2015), generating momentum for CPM licensure. Currently, 33 states license CPMs (NACPM 2020), including a gain of 7 states over the last five years. NACPM provides direction and tools to CPM advocates as well as technical support to state legislators and regulators. NACPM has become a trusted source of leadership and support that state advocates turn to with increasing frequency.

Federal Policy

Securing federal recognition for CPMs, an NACPM priority since 2009, is a linchpin for all health professionals and key to consumer access. It will be achieved by amending the Social Security Act, which houses the Medicare and Medicaid laws, to mandate federal Medicaid reimbursement for CPM services. In addition, this policy will open doors for inclusion in the systems of care, health professional education, and reimbursement that typically support health professions.

Workforce development is a key NACPM policy priority. In 2019, I led NACPM's efforts to help secure the introduction of two pieces of legislation to provide the first-ever federal funding for midwifery education. The Midwives for Maximizing Optimal Maternal Outcomes (MOMS) Act (NACPM 2019a) will create new permanent funding programs for midwifery education within the Public Health Service Act. Also, as a result of legislation passed in December 2019, CPM-accredited schools are now eligible to apply for HRSA grants for the Scholarships for Disadvantaged Students Program. Federal funding, a staple for decades for physicians and nurses, will address the perinatal workforce shortage, bring urgently needed care to families in provider-shortage areas, both rural and urban, and support more midwives of color to join the profession.

NACPM engages with federal agencies to promote the inclusion of CPMs in our systems of care. We have provided technical assistance to the CMS for the implementation of provisions of the Affordable Care Act that impact birth centers. Recently, we were invited to consult with the Center for

Medicare and Medicaid Innovation on strategies for including CPMs in demonstration models to test new payment and service delivery models.

The Path Forward

Over the last two decades, NACPM has increasingly led on leveraging health policy to benefit childbearing people. I have built key relationships on NACPM's behalf with state and national health leaders and policy makers that are expanding and augmenting NACPM's influence. NACPM is now regularly invited to consult with members of Congress and, at times, with federal agencies on the development of perinatal legislation and policies and to collaborate with other health professional organizations on national initiatives. In part due to our efforts, policy makers are finally turning appropriate attention to addressing the urgent needs of childbearing people. It is an exciting journey to be on, discovering and leveraging the power of ordinary everyday committed midwives to influence systems that have such profound impact on the lives of childbearing people and to experience what it takes to evolve into effective leaders in the policy sphere.

References

ACNM, MANA, and NACPM. 2013. "Supporting Healthy and Normal Physiologic Childbirth: A Consensus Statement by ACNM, MANA, and NACPM." *Journal of Perinatal Education* 22(1): 14–18. https://doi.org/10.1891/1058-1243.22.1.14.

Cheyney, M., M. Bovbjerg, C. Everson, W. Gordon, D. Hannibal, and S. Vedam. 2014. "Outcomes of Care for 16,924 Planned Home Births in the United States: The Midwives Alliance of North America Statistics Project, 2004 to 2009." *Journal of Midwifery & Women's Health* 59(1): 17–27. https://doi.org/10.1111/jmwh.12172.

Health Management Associates. 2007. "Midwifery Licensure and Discipline Program in Washington State: Economic

Costs and Benefits." October 31. https://www.nacpm.org /documents/Midwifery_Cost_Study_10-31-07.pdf.

The Lancet. 2014. "Midwifery: An Executive Summary for *The Lancet's* Series." https://www.thelancet.com/pb/assets/raw /Lancet/stories/series/midwifery/midwifery_exec_summ.pdf.

National Association of Certified Professional Midwives (NACPM). 2017. "CPMs: Midwifery Landscape and Future Directions: A Set of Briefing Papers and Recommendations." October. https://www.nacpm.org/wp -content/uploads/2017/10/2A1-CPMs_What-We-Have -Learned-Why-Our-Practice-is-Critical.pdf.

National Association of Certified Professional Midwives (NACPM). 2019a. "Legislation to Fund Midwifery Education Introduced in the U.S. House of Representatives." August 5. https://nacpm.org/legislation-to-fund-midwifery -education-introduced-in-the-u-s-house-of-representatives/.

National Association of Certified Professional Midwives (NACPM). 2019b. "$2.5 Million to Educate Disadvantaged Student Midwives Becomes Law." December. https://nacpm.org/2-5-million-to-educate -disadvantaged-student-midwives-becomes-law/.

National Association of Certified Professional Midwives (NACPM). 2020. "Legal Recognition of CPMs." May 15. https://nacpm.org/about-cpms/who-are-cpms/legal -recognition-of-cpms/.

Sakala, C., and M. P. Corry. 2008. *Evidence-Based Maternity Care, What It Is and What It Can Achieve.* New York: Milbank Memorial Fund. https://www.milbank.org /wp-content/uploads/2016/04/0809MaternityCare.pdf.

United States Midwifery Education, Regulation, and Association (US MERA). 2015. "Principles for Model US Midwifery Legislation & Regulation." November 20. http://www.usmera.org/index.php/2015/11/20/principles -for-model-u-s-midwifery-legislation-regulation/.

United States Midwifery Education, Regulation, and
Association (US MERA). n.d. Homepage. http://www
.usmera.org/.

Visionary Vanguard Group. 2017. "The JJ Way: Community-
Based Maternity Center: Final Evaluation Report." http://
www.commonsensechildbirth.org/wp-content/uploads
/2019/07/The-JJ-Way%C2%AE-Community-based
-Maternity-Center-Evaluation-Report-2017-1.pdf.

Washington State Health Care Authority. 2016.
"Reimbursement for Births Performed at Birth Center."
October. https://www.hca.wa.gov/assets/program
/2eshb-2376-birth-centers.pdf.

*Mary Lawlor, CPM, LM, has been in home birth practice in south-
ern New England since 1981 and opened the Monadnock Birth
Center in New Hampshire in 2008. She is a passionate advocate
for midwives and for women's access to the care of midwives and a
national leader in shaping the public policy agenda for the NACPM
in support of these goals. She participated in the successful initiative
to license CPMs in Vermont and New Hampshire in 2000 and has
served as an adviser to the Vermont Office of Professional Regulation since 2002, helping to oversee the practice of midwifery in the
state. In 2000, she became a founder of the NACPM and served
as president from 2002 until 2012 before becoming the executive
director in 2012. She serves as a national midwifery policy adviser
to the NACPM, which includes advocating to the U.S. Congress
and federal agencies for increased access for women across the country to CPM services and high-quality, high-value maternity care.*

Equity in Midwifery
Indra Wood Lusero

I was a queer polyamorous twentysomething in the late 1990s,
and my college girlfriend and I had decided to make babies
with our gay college roommate. He would not "just" be a sperm

donor but a coparent, and we would forge a pathway into family unlike any we knew. We would both get pregnant, and she would go first because her parents were more likely to reject the plan—the thinking being that a grandbaby might soften them to the queerness of it all and make it harder for them to reject their second grandbaby once I gave birth (it worked!).

At the same time, I was finishing grad school, working at a flower shop, and performing my one-person show. I thought about power dynamics a lot. I thought about marginalization and discrimination and majorities and minorities and how societies change. In high school, I was recognized as a "champion of the underdog," and these were the same themes in my show. It turns out, these themes are my life's work.

After going to college in the Northwest, I was excited to move back to Colorado, where I felt so rooted to the land my ancestors had inhabited for generations. Ancestors on my dad's side come from northern New Mexico/southern Colorado which had been the land of many tribes (Ute, Apache, Pueblo Indians), a Spanish colony, part of Mexico, and finally part of the United States. I was acutely aware of being from a small lineage of people who, over hundreds of years in this region, had been both colonizer and colonized.

There was just over a year between when my first son was born and when I got pregnant, and during that time, I started reading *Our Word Is Our Weapon*, a collection of writings by Subcomandante Marcos, a spokesperson of the Zapatistas. The Zapatista uprising involved a community of mainly Indigenous people in the Mexican state of Chiapas who took up arms and mobilized the imagination against powerful corporate landowners backed by multinational corporations. It was an inspiring story about the underdog's innate resourcefulness and drive for equity.

Skipping perhaps the best part of the story (Kailey 2007), after I gave birth at home with a beautiful team of midwives, I was captivated by the treasure trove of power and energy that felt available to me because of that experience. I marveled at how little technology my labor required, especially in comparison to my elder son's hospital birth. I marveled at how easy it was to imagine every birthing person having such care regardless of their station in life. It felt revolutionary. It felt like a Zapatista uprising: small, but mighty, powerful enough to ignite the world and fundamentally redistribute resources more equitably.

That is my vision. I truly believe that if every birthing person had access to fully supportive midwifery care, in the Midwives Model of Care (National Association of Certified Professional Midwives (NACPM) 2008), it would change the world, it would make the world a more equitable and just place. The Midwives Model of Care assumes that pregnancy and birth are normal life processes and that "physical, psychological, and social well-being" matter throughout the childbearing cycle (NACPM 2008). The model is about providing "individualized education, counseling, and prenatal care, continuous hands-on assistance during labor and delivery, and postpartum support," while "minimizing technological interventions," and referring people to obstetrical care as needed (NACPM 2008).

It does not sound like too much to ask. But as it turns out, not enough people have access to this kind of care, both in the United States (Vedam et al. 2018) and all over the world (UNFPA, ICM, and WHO 2014) . In the United States, only about 9 percent of births are attended by a midwife (Martin et al. 2019), and for many, maternity care in general is inaccessible, inadequate, and inequitable (Sakala 2020). Perhaps most starkly, Native and Black people are two and three times *more likely to die* as a result of pregnancy than white people (Sakala 2020). Access to quality care varies by region, rural versus urban, and even varies between hospitals in the same city.

It is not too much to ask, and it is not too expensive to implement; however, it does require a reordering of power and priorities. Across time and culture, the relationship between midwifery and society mirrors the relationship between women and society. In recent history, and especially in the history of the United States over the last 200 years, this has meant that midwives in the United States and its tribes and territories were marginalized.

Indeed, so few people are cared for by midwives in this country today because physicians sought to eliminate them altogether 100 years ago (Rooks 1997). They did so using overtly sexist, racist, anti-immigrant, and classist language (Rooks 1997), which had a disproportionate effect on birthing people from marginalized communities as well as the midwives and potential midwives from those communities. Today, the relatively small midwifery workforce in the United State is, not surprisingly, mostly white.

Given the role that bias plays in health care, homogenizing health care providers so that they mainly represent only some of us (and poorly at that) has dramatic (and dramatically inequitable) consequences—consequences quite similar to those experienced by the Zapatistas due to the consolidation of power on behalf of corporations by governments, coordinating not for the common good but for the good of the few. Notably, sometimes those coordinating for the few use words that suggest the public good despite having motivations that are not entirely grounded in the public good.

This is one of the lessons I have learned from the history of midwifery and childbirth. Indeed, the American anti-midwife campaign of the twentieth century purported to be about health and safety, as did the experimentation of Dr. J. Marion Simms on enslaved women without anesthesia in the nineteenth century. Many "maternal health" efforts throughout history have failed to be grounded in the health and safety of *all* (Roberts 1997; Ross and Solinger 2017).

When I chose to birth at home as someone from multiple minority communities, I did not know this history. But I did know that my great-grandmother on my dad's side was a *curandera* and community worker; and I knew that a great-aunt on my mom's side was a midwife; and, most importantly, I knew that my mom had given birth to my two youngest siblings at home (I was there!). I knew that dominant society did not always have *me* or nondominant people in mind, so I would have to take what was useful and leave what was harmful to thrive. And that is what I did, as many of us do.

But instead of learning to cope with being the "other" in a society not made for us, it is time that we create a society that could actually work well for all of us. This is equity, the organization of things so that they work well for all. Ensuring that everyone has access to the Midwives Model of Care is one way to help bring about just such a world; "The world with the many worlds that the world needs," as the Zapatistas might say. We can and should strive to bring about a more equitable world, so that "humanity, recognizing itself to be plural, different, inclusive, tolerant of itself, full of hope, continues" (Marcos and DeLeon 2001).

References

Kailey, M., ed. 2007. *Focus on the Fabulous: Colorado GLBT Voices*, 141–144. Boulder: Johnson Books (Note: My birth story, "Luminaria," is published under my former name, L. Lusero, in this collection.)

Marcos, S., and J. P. DeLeon, eds. 2001. *Our Word Is Our Weapon: Selected Writings*. New York: Seven Stories Press.

Martin, J. A., B. E. Hamilton, M. J. K. S. Osterman, A. K. Driscoll, and T. J. Mathews. 2019. "Births: Final Data for 2018." *National Vital Statistics Reports* 68, no. 13. https://www.cdc.gov/nchs/data/nvsr/nvsr68/nvsr68_13-508.pdf.

National Association of Certified Professional Midwives (NACPM). 2008. "Midwives Model of Care." https://nacpm.org/about-cpms/midwifery-model-of-care/.

Roberts, D. 1997. *Killing the Black Body: Race, Reproduction and the Meaning of Liberty*. New York: Random House.

Rooks, J. P. 1997. *Midwifery and Childbirth in America*. Philadelphia: Temple University Press.

Ross, L. J., and R. Solinger. 2017. *Reproductive Justice: An Introduction*. Berkeley: University of California Press.

Sakala, C. 2020. *Maternity Care in the United States: We Can—And Must—Do Better*. Issue Brief, February. Washington, DC: National Partnership for Women & Families. https://www.nationalpartnership.org/our-work /resources/healthcare/maternity-care-in-the-united.pdf.

UNFPA, ICM, and WHO. 2014. *The State of the World's Midwifery 2014: A Universal Pathway. A Women's Right to Health*. New York: United Nations Population Fund. https://www.unfpa.org/sowmy.

Vedam, S., K. Stoll, M. MacDorman, E. Declercq, R. Cramer, M. Cheyney, T. Fisher, et al. 2018. "Mapping Integration of Midwives across the United States: Impact on Access, Equity, and Outcomes." *PLoS One* 13(2): e0192523. https://doi.org/10.1371/journal.pone.0192523.

Indra Wood Lusero is a queer, Latinx birth justice attorney and parent who loves to tackle new territory, dive into cutting-edge issues and ideas, and navigate periods of change and uncertainty. Indra is the founder of Elephant Circle and the Birth Rights Bar Association and a staff attorney at the National Advocates for Pregnant Women. Indra recently spearheaded the creation of "Birth Rights: A Resource for Everyday People to Defend Human Rights during Labor and Birth."

Labor and Postpartum Doula Support: How Doulas Help the Transitions of Pregnancy, Childbirth, and the Postpartum Time and Why They Are Important
Kristy Zadrozny

Doulas are an essential element of the perinatal health care system. The doula profession may be an emerging field, but the role a doula plays is an ancient one. A doula is an emotional, informational, and physical support person during pregnancy, childbirth, and the early postpartum time. A doula's primary work is to provide continuous, nonjudgmental support as a new family goes through this transformational time. Historically, this role belonged to sisters, friends, aunties, and female neighbors, a familiar person who had experienced the birth process before. Today, in the United States, women are giving birth later in life, and they may be moving to new cities and countries, without an immediate support network available (Mathews and Hamilton 2002). Professional doulas emerged to fill in this role when family and friends could not.

Additionally, with industrialization, the culture of birth changed. Women began giving birth in hospitals, with obstetricians rather than their neighborhood midwife. The move to hospital-based birth had some benefits for women and babies. This move also meant more interventions in healthy pregnancies, which increased risks for both mom and baby. Some women experienced a feeling of disconnection from the birth process. Disconnection from childbirth contributed to feelings of fear, anxiety, and apprehension surrounding the process. Feeling safe and secure during childbirth reduces the need for interventions and allows the birth process to unfold ordinarily, which is safer for both the birthing person and the baby (Lothian 2009).

The Role of the Doula

Why would someone need a doula when they have obstetricians, midwives, and nurses caring for them? A doula's role is not clinical at all, which is what makes it so crucial for the birth process. A clinical care provider has an essential job: keeping mom and baby safe and healthy. A doula's job is to make sure that mom, partner, and baby are feeling happy and satisfied. Ideally, the clinical care provider and doula work together collaboratively with the birth family as their guide. Research tells us that women and babies have better birth outcomes when they feel emotionally supported during the birth process (Kozhimannil et al. 2013). A client-centered approach means that the pregnant person not only understands the birth process but also plans and outlines her birth preferences for her care provider. Many women find that preparing a birth plan is helpful, as it creates a road map for them and their care provider to be on the same page; this opens communication channels and creates a common ground for discussion. A good birth plan lists the five or six things that are most important to a family. It is important to remember that a birth plan is not set in stone, as we cannot control the birth process, but we can be active participants in the decisions that take place along the way.

Pregnancy, childbirth, and parenting a newborn person are the most significant transitions a family will go through in their lifetime. Transitions can be exciting, overwhelming, and sometimes scary. Childbirth is a little bit like learning to walk, teething, or going through puberty. Sure, the body usually figures out how to do it all out on its own, but there are moments when this kind of growth and change can feel uncomfortable. As humans, we sometimes need extra help to get through those uncomfortable moments. Support comes in many forms; there is hand-holding, a comforting back rub, or someone to prepare a nourishing meal. Other times, support is in the form of emotional support; it is having someone remind you that everything is unfolding just as it should. There is nothing shameful or strange about it. Humans grow in these moments of discomfort; we rely on our support networks as guides. Our support networks help through our most challenging moments; this builds confidence in ourselves and feelings of self-reliance to get through future challenges.

In childbirth, there is a hormone called oxytocin that makes the uterus contract, which helps to open the cervix, which is the exit for the baby. As it turns out, we also make oxytocin when we are cuddling with a loved one, breastfeeding our babies, getting a massage, having an orgasm, or falling in love. These joyful feelings do not always bubble up when we are hanging out in a hospital! A doula and other support people can help create a supportive environment not only in labor but in the weeks leading up to birth for optimal oxytocin production.

Change and Stress

We all know that change can be hard. One of the most significant changes that happen in a person's life is going from being an autonomous person to being pregnant to then becoming a parent. Changing bodies, changing relationships, and changing identities bring a lot of questions and potential stressors. Stress impedes the birth process by blocking oxytocin production. We can start to understand the importance of having someone like a doula to help us to reduce stress and make these changes a lot more manageable. The practice of asking for help during pregnancy establishes a healthy habit of seeking out support when challenges arise in the future. Asking for help is an integral part of parenting.

Doula as Identity

Many doulas find a calling into the profession from their own childbirth experience. Others have witnessed someone close to them give birth. Furthermore, a doula that has not had any children of her own can still feel called to support the birth process because she understands how it feels to go through other kinds of transitions and wants to support women as they go through theirs. The empathy that arises in us, from our own harrowing experiences, can be the vehicle for stepping into the role of a doula. Many doulas are doulas long before they do their initial training. Perhaps you are the kind of person who notices when someone else is uncomfortable, or perhaps you find that your friends and family call upon you in times of need. Typically, a doula is great at holding her center, especially when things are stressful. A doula can hold space in the most profound sense. Holding space can look like organizing the logistics of any situation, helping others to keep calm, and helping everyone to move through whatever is arising.

A doula gives a lot of herself to help others, so the doula needs to make time to do things that bring her joy. We are our best selves when we feel nourished, well rested, and happy. Maintaining healthy boundaries is an essential part of being a doula.

Where It All Begins

Childbirth is the beginning of all life. We are all born from our mothers, and we grow within a family system that creates our identities, which shapes us into our adult selves. There is an incredible need for women to hold and support each other through this process. We can hold the *doula ethic* within our hearts and minds when supporting our dear ones through the childbirth process or any transitional period in life.

What Is the Doula Ethic?

A doula does not have an agenda; first and foremost, she supports the birthing family's wishes. A doula is nonjudgmental; she has an open and loving mindset. A doula is attuned to her own needs and asks for help when she needs it, to be fully in service of another.

Many people believe that a doula is an advocate for her clients, when, in fact, her role is more as an ally and coach. A key thing to remember is that when we speak for others, we take away their agency; a doula instead gives her clients the information and tools to speak for themselves. These are skills they will carry into parenthood.

A doula's goal is to help her clients feel self-assured in their ability to care for their new babies, and the new baby then feels loved and protected. A feeling of safety and security in a baby is the foundation of building secure attachments between parents and their children (Shorey 2015).

Do You Want to Become a Doula?

There are many routes toward professional certification, so it is necessary to explore the different certifying bodies to find the one that resonates with you. When researching certifying bodies, it is essential to understand who is doing the training and what the process of certification entails for the particular organization. Generally speaking, certification requires a 20-hour in-person training followed by a comprehensive exam that focuses on the doula's role in the birth process or postpartum time. You will need to attend actual births and work with postpartum families to complete your certification. Most organizations give two years to conclude this process. There is no traditional path to becoming a doula, so it is important to recognize that you will be learning on the job. The first few client cases will be opportunities to give back to one's community by volunteering or offering services at a reduced fee.

Once certified, many doulas round out their service offerings by taking additional certification classes in complementary skills, such as hands-on massage, optimal fetal positioning, aromatherapy, or lactation counseling. The opportunities for growth are abundant, and with dedication, it is possible to carve out a fulfilling career as a doula.

References

Kozhimannil, K. B., R. R. Hardeman, L. B. Attanasio, C. Blauer-Peterson, and M. O'Brien. 2013. "Doula Care, Birth Outcomes, and Costs among Medicaid Beneficiaries." *American Journal of Public Health* 103: e113–e121. https://doi.org/10.2105/AJPH.2012.301201.

Lothian, J. A. 2009. "Safe, Healthy Birth: What Every Pregnant Woman Needs to Know." *Journal of Perinatal Education* 18(3): 48–54. https://doi.org/10.1624/105812409X461225.

Mathews, T. J., and B. E. Hamilton. 2002. "Mean Age of Mother, 1970–2000." *National Vital Statistics Reports* 51, no. 1. Hyattsville, MD: National Center for Health Statistics. https://www.cdc.gov/nchs/data/nvsr/nvsr51/nvsr51_01.pdf.

Shorey, H. 2015. "The Keys to Rewarding Relationships: Secure Attachment." *Psychology Today* online, February 12. https://www.psychologytoday.com/us/blog/the-freedom -change/201502/the-keys-rewarding-relationships-secure -attachment.

Kristy Zadrozny is a New York City–based educator and seasoned labor doula. She teaches new and expecting parents, as well as the professional doulas that support them, mindfulness-based theory and practice and family relationship dynamics as it applies to the perinatal period. She is New York State's resident labor and post-partum doula faculty member for the Childbirth and Postpartum Professional Association.

Gender and Consumption
Alec Cali

In the last decade, the United States has experienced a new form of celebrating incoming children and gift items necessary for the baby's first few months. Baby showers have historically been a celebration of coming motherhood and the child, and they were relatively gender neutral in the celebration of the baby (Paoletti 2012). Items gifted at the party tended to deal with androgynous child necessities, such as diapers or strollers. The increased importance of gendering children as early as possible, partly to fuel the growth of gender-reveal parties, over the last decades has begun reinforcing gender norms much sooner for children and parents alike. In the first several weeks of pregnancy, the fetus is largely ignored: an at-home pregnancy test confirms the parents' suspicions, and the subsequent physicians' appointments quickly guide the pregnant person in how best to be healthy during the pregnancy. Physicians often begin making gendered health recommendations during pregnancy after the blood tests, and ultrasounds that happen between week 14 and week 18 (Nissim 2019). While the blood tests and ultrasounds continue during the pregnancy, the sex determination is important not only for how physicians change their treatment of a fetus but also for how parents begin treating their future child.

Although the designation of *male* or *female* is given at this critical point in a patient's obstetric care, it is not because the physicians believe it serves a clinical purpose. Few families are at risk of the genetic diseases that sex determination is required to manage, with almost all parents receiving a sex determination test doing so for no clinical benefit (Gharekhanloo 2018). Instead, physicians schedule sex determination ultrasounds at this time because it is the earliest it is medically possible for such determinations to be done (Samuels 2018). Despite medicine's desire to utilize clinically insignificant tests, physicians often fail to explain to parents that ultrasounds are inaccurate in determining genitalia about 10 percent of the time (Manzanares et al. 2016). Similarly, practitioners often fail to explain to parents that genitalia is not the only measure of biologic sex, a person's gender identity is not determined at birth, or that a person's gender identity is not linked to their biologic sex. Despite these limitations, parents often receive the sex of their child as a medical fact and accept it as their child's gender. The determination of the fetal sex is important for several reasons, including the signification of the fetus's existence to the parents beyond a mass of cells and the medically sanctioned enforcement of gender norms starting in pregnancy.

The rise of baby showers as a popular way to celebrate an incoming child has quickly been followed by new lines of party supplies, companies created entirely to coordinate gender-reveal parties, rapid internet viewership changes, and millions of dollars in damages being done from parties (Pesce 2019; Schiller 2019; Gender Reveal Cakery 2020; Rosenblatt 2018; Party City 2020). While there is little research on whether gender-reveal parties are fully replacing baby showers as a tradition, the gendering of a child in the womb is becoming part of America's pregnancy ritual (Pasche Guignard 2015). Although parents receive incomplete counseling on the sex determination received from their practitioner, many use this information as one of the first real ways to relate to and describe their unborn children (Carter 2010). This attempt to describe and relate to their unborn child is not isolated, however; it interacts with the ideas they hold and those marketed by media and commercial venues (Berger 1972).

It would be a mistake to say that children's products before the advent of the gender reveal were androgynous, but products purchased for preparation of childbirth were relatively neutral. Strollers, cribs, baby formula, paint for nursery, basic toys, pacifiers, socks, and clothes could all be bought without knowing a baby's gender—and without making the baby "gender bend" in an offensive way (Paoletti 2012). With the medical prescription of gender, parents, friends, and family are better equipped to begin preparing for the baby by purchasing the correctly gendered items. This is made easy by the ocean of powder blue and pink items, trucks, and princess-themed baby clothes that are available for purchase, including toilets for potty training (BuyBuyBaby 2020). Gender-reveal parties require a purposeful purchase of these gendered items, although it could be argued that the pink toilet was the only one available at the time.

To successfully announce the gender, the party must be planned around stereotypes: if you cut a cake, pop a balloon, shoot a barrel, or cut into lasagna, you will see blue or pink to state the gender of the fetus, now baby (Dellatto 2019; Schiller 2019; Rosenblatt 2018). If the wrong color icing is used, the gender reveal quite literally fails. There should be no excuse to dress a baby incorrectly, buy the wrong toys, or paint their room wrong if you know the baby's gender. We often see explanations for gender-reveal parties that include desiring to know which gendered items to buy the child, rather than hoping for a boy or girl (Schiller 2019; Pasche Guignard 2015).

Parents often purchase baby products, maternity products, guidebooks, health products, and lifestyle subscriptions in preparation of their child to relate to their baby and to express their own gender roles (Clarke 2004). While deciding on what products to purchase during pregnancy and even before pregnancy, we see the expectations of parents' gender identity become reinforced through expected purchases recommended by physicians, ads, and family members. Women, regardless of their intent to have a child, are frequently expected to prepare for pregnancy early on in their life by maintaining or improving their health (Waggoner 2017).

Women frequently demonstrate these forms of consumptive womanhood and intended motherhood by purchasing the correct medical, food, and parenting products and planning children's events such as baby showers and gender-reveal parties (Dow 2019; Hays 1998; Reich 2016). Physicians often ask women to make purchasing decisions well in advance of a consumer's reproductive plans, using consumer choice to mold the consumer-patient to gender norms—asking them to purchase specific vitamins despite not having a deficiency, asking them to buy different foods and attend a gym (to prepare for potential pregnancy, not because weight is a health issue), and recommending frequent check-ins with their physicians to ensure their health is optimal (Waggoner 2017). Women are often required to make the vast majority of decisions related to child-related purchases and decisions on matters related to pregnancy, with the women who are best able to make such purchases and decisions lauded as the "best" mothers (Hays 1998; Reich 2016; Dow 2019).

Unfortunately, many women are unable to afford, both financially and with time, the high levels of consumption required to properly gender themselves and their baby. Women are least likely to hold jobs that provide benefits such as paid time off, childcare, or health insurance (Collins 2019; Block and Subramanian 2015). Black and brown women also have experienced higher rates of medical malpractice, are more likely to live in food deserts, or work jobs that provide low pay and no benefits (Damaske 2011; Washington 2006). When women are unable to make the necessary purchases and lifestyle choices to prepare for their child and motherhood, they are frequently criticized by their physician, media, and family (Reich 2016; Waggoner 2017; Damaske 2011). This is heightened for Black and brown women and low-income women, especially low-income Black and brown women, who not only face direct criticism but run the risk of having Child Protective Services called if they do not sufficiently subscribe to gender and parenting norms (Roberts 2002, 2017; Rose 2015).

While many families use sex determinations to better relate to their incoming child and further solidify parental roles and gender norms, many are left out of the ideal because of structural issues (Dow 2019). Despite their love for the incoming child, financial and consumption constraints caused by decades of public policy decisions frequently make it difficult for women and parents to successfully consume gender for their baby or themselves—allowing state agencies such as Child Protective Services to prosecute them for insufficiently preparing for their child (Massey and Denton 1993; Roberts 2002). Although it is important for parents to relate to their children in ways that are significant to themselves, purchasing gender norms in pregnancy has created a series of unequal events, where some children and parents can never completely buy their identity because of circumstances beyond their control. We must begin reducing our emphasis on consuming gender to ensure that parents and children are able to freely express their gender identities without fear of stigma or persecution.

References

Berger, J. 1972. *Ways of Seeing*. London: Penguin Books.

Block, Jason P., and S. V. Subramanian. 2015. "Moving beyond 'Food Deserts': Reorienting United States Policies to Reduce Disparities in Diet Quality." *PLoS Medicine* 12(12). https://doi.org/10.1371/journal.pmed.1001914.

BuyBuyBaby. 2020. "Summer Infant My Size Potty in Pink." https://www.buybuybaby.com/store/product/summer-infant-reg-my-size-potty-in-pink/1061563063.

Carter, S. K. 2010. "Beyond Control: Body and Self in Women's Childbearing Narratives." *Sociology of Health & Illness* 32(7): 993–1009. https://doi.org/10.1111/j.1467-9566.2010.01261.x.

Clarke, A. J. 2004. "Maternity and Materiality: Becoming a Mother in Consumer Culture." In *Consuming Motherhood,* edited by J. Taylor and L. Layne, 55–71. Princeton, NJ: Rutgers University Press.

Collins, C. 2019. *Making Motherhood Work: How Women Manage Careers and Caregiving.* Princeton, NJ: Princeton University Press.

Damaske, S. 2011. *For the Family? How Class and Gender Shape Women's Work.* New York: Oxford University Press.

Dellatto, M. 2019. "Lasagna Is the Gross New Way to Reveal Your Baby's Gender." *New York Post,* January 22. https://nypost.com/2019/01/22/lasagna-is-the-gross-new-way-to-reveal-your-babys-gender/.

Dow, D. M. 2019. *Mothering while Black: Boundaries and Burdens of Middle-Class Parenthood.* Oakland: University of California Press.

Gender Reveal Cakery. 2020. "Gender Reveal Cakes—New York City." http://genderrevealcakery.com/.

Gharekhanloo, F. 2018. "The Ultrasound Identification of Fetal Gender at the Gestational Age of 11–12 Weeks." *Journal of Family Medicine and Primary Care* 7(1): 210–212. https://doi.org/10.4103/jfmpc.jfmpc_180_17.

Hays, S. 1998. *The Cultural Contradictions of Motherhood.* New Haven, CT: Yale University Press.

Manzanares, S., A. Benítez, M. Naveiro-Fuentes, M. S. López-Criado, and M. Sánchez-Gila. 2016. "Accuracy of

Fetal Sex Determination on Ultrasound Examination in the First Trimester of Pregnancy: Fetal Sex Determination in First Trimester." *Journal of Clinical Ultrasound* 44(5): 272–277. https://doi.org/10.1002/jcu.22320.

Massey, D. S., and N. A. Denton. 19933. *American Apartheid: Segregation and the Making of the Underclass.* Cambridge, MA: Harvard University Press.

Nissim, J. 2019. Interview with Julie Nissim. In-person. July 23, 2009, interviewer's name: Alec Cali.

Paoletti, J. B. 2012. *Pink and Blue: Telling the Boys from the Girls in America.* Bloomington: Indiana University Press.

Party City. 2020. "Party City: 'Big Reveal Gender Reveal Supplies.'" https://www.partycity.com/big-reveal-gender-reveal.

Pasche Guignard, F. 2015. "A Gendered Bun in the Oven. The Gender-Reveal Party as a New Ritualization during Pregnancy." *Studies in Religion/Sciences Religieuses* 44(4): 479–500. https://doi.org/10.1177/0008429815599802.

Pesce, N. L. 2019. "The Mom behind the Gender-Reveal Craze Now Asks, 'Who Cares What Gender the Baby Is?'" MarketWatch, July 29. https://www.marketwatch.com/story/the-mom-behind-the-gender-reveal-craze-now-asks-who-cares-what-gender-the-baby-is-2019-07-29.

Reich, J. A. 2016. *Calling the Shots: Why Parents Reject Vaccines.* New York: New York University Press.

Roberts, D. E. 2002. *Shattered Bonds: The Color of Child Welfare.* New York: Basic Books.

Roberts, D. E. 2017. *Killing the Black Body: Race, Reproduction, and the Meaning of Liberty.* 2nd ed. New York: Vintage Books.

Rose, R. 2015. "Single Mom Leaves Kids in Food Court to Go on Interview Nearby, Gets Arrested for Abandoning Them." *Cosmopolitan*, July 20. https://www.cosmopolitan.com/politics/news/a43557/single-mom-arrested-for

-abandoning-kids-during-job-interview-even-though-they
-were-30-feet-away/.

Rosenblatt, K. 2018. "Video Released of Gender Reveal That
Sparked Arizona's Sawmill Fire." NBC News, November
27. https://www.nbcnews.com/news/us-news/u-s-forest
-service-releases-video-arizona-gender-reveal-sparked
-n940506.

Samuels, E. 2018. "How Do Parents Find Out the Sex
of Their Baby Today? Exploring the Trend of Gender-
Reveal Parties." *Washington Post*, May 13. https://www
.washingtonpost.com/news/parenting/wp/2018/05/13/how
-do-parents-find-out-the-sex-of-their-baby-today-exploring
-the-new-trend-of-gender-reveal-parties/.

Schiller, R. 2019. "Why the Mother Who Started Gender-
Reveal Parties Regrets Them." *The Guardian*, October 20.
https://www.theguardian.com/lifeandstyle/2019/oct/20
/why-the-mother-who-started-gender-reveal-parties-regrets
-them.

Waggoner, M. 2017. *The Zero Trimester*. Oakland: University
of California Press.

Washington, H. 2006. *Medical Apartheid*. New York: Harlem
Moon/Random House.

*Alec Cali is a PhD student at Stony Brook University and is
researching the anti-vaccination movement. They are interested in
how vaccine skeptics bridge parenting ideals with the ideals surrounding proper medical care. Alec's research incorporates compu-
tational methods, cultural criticism, and economic analysis.*

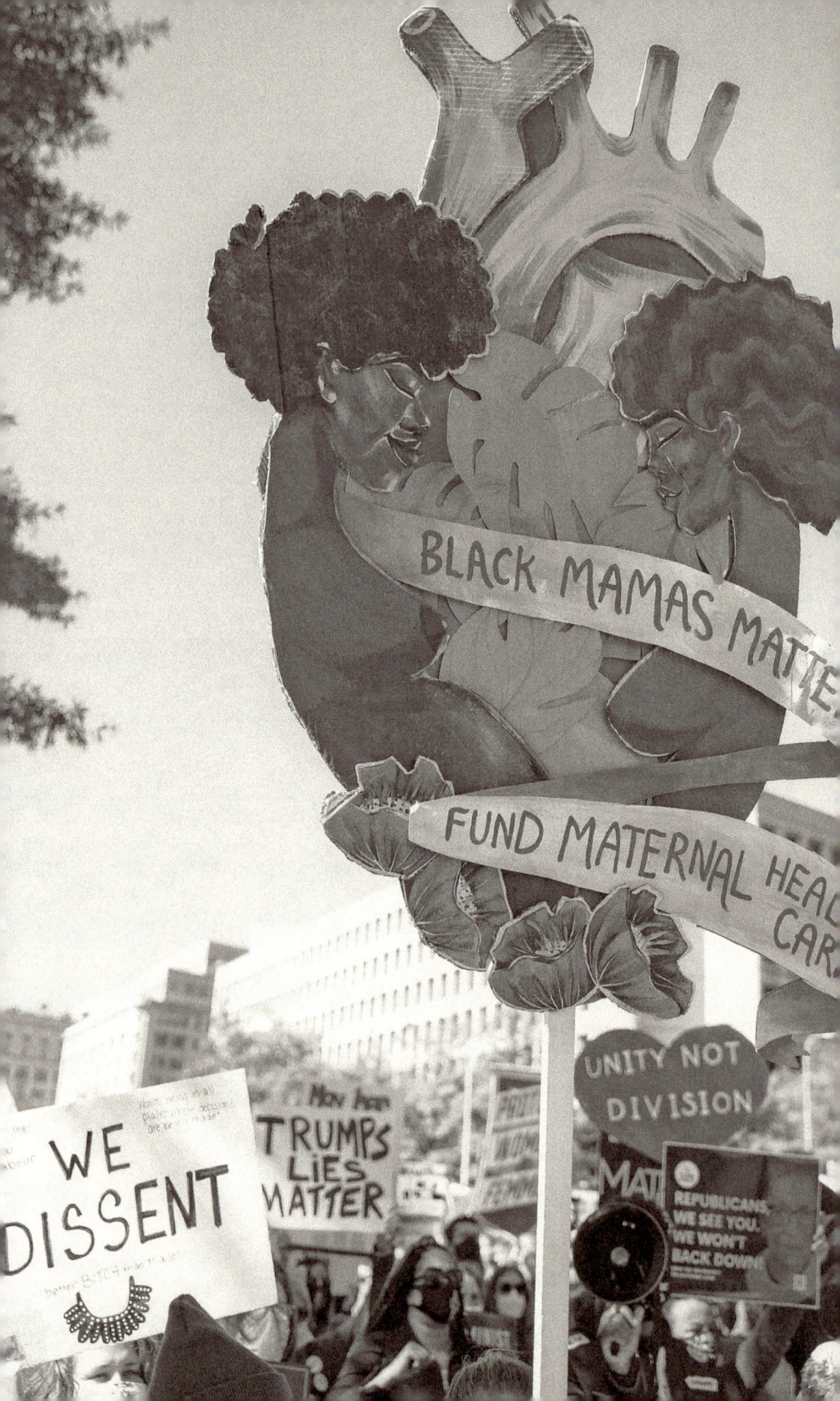

This chapter contains brief profiles of individuals and organizations who are important to understanding pregnancy and birth in the United States and how we have come to view these important life events. There are, of course, many more people and organizations that could have been included. We honor the work of birth and Reproductive Justice workers everywhere.

People, General

Apgar, Virginia (1909–1974)

Virginia Apgar received her medical degree in the 1930s, at a point when women were around 5 percent of all physicians. She had wanted to become a surgeon, but those options were even fewer for women. Anesthesiology was just starting to develop as a medical specialty, and so opportunities for women were somewhat more open. She eventually headed the Division of Anesthesiology at Columbia University, in New York, the first woman there to achieve the position of full professor.

At that point in the medical management of childbirth and infant care, it was standard for people to be fully anesthetized at the moment of birth. This meant that newborn babies were also fully anesthetized. The popular cultural image of a physician holding the baby upside down just after birth,

Reproductive Justice activism. (Julian Leshay/Dreamstime.com)

and the laboring person strapped down on a table, while "spanking" the baby into consciousness comes from this practice: unanesthetized infants do not sleep through being born. Babies were sent off to newborn nurseries and mothers to recovery rooms.

Apgar was concerned with the condition of these babies and improving their health and survival. She saw that it was important to distinguish the babies who were fundamentally well, though temporarily anesthetized, from those who were in trouble. In 1952, Apgar developed a 5-point score to assess the health of the baby immediately at birth. The points to be assessed are (1) skin tone—without oxygen, a bluish tone indicates a problem; (2) pulse rate; (3) reflexes; (4) muscle tone; and (5) respiration. This can be done very quickly by whomever is attending the birth.

In 1963, this scoring system became known as the *APGAR score* with a clever acronym: appearance, for the skin tone; pulse; grimace, for the irritability of the reflex response; activity, for muscle tone; and respiration. The APGAR score has become standard in birth management.

Virginia Apgar went on to work at the March of Dimes, as vice president of medical affairs, and helped move that organization into its concern with congenital disabilities and their prevention. She was responsible for a campaign for immunization against rubella (German measles), which if a woman has during pregnancy can have serious outcomes for the baby.

Apgar was an important figure in drawing attention to the health of babies. In addition to her many (over 70) academic publications on anesthesiology, newborn resuscitation, and congenital disabilities, she wrote (with coauthor Joan Beck) the book *Is My Baby All Right?* for the more general audience of parents.

Callen, Maude E. (1898–1990)

It is through the life and work of Maude E. Callen that the term *nurse-midwife* was introduced to the American public, along with some awareness of midwifery's role in the African American communities of the South.

Callen was born one of thirteen sisters and was orphaned by the age of six. Her uncle, a physician named William J Gunn, brought her into his home. In the early twentieth century, Black physicians were, of course, extraordinarily rare, and his story is itself interesting; he began his career as a driver for a white physician who mentored and supported him through medical school. As an African American woman, it was probably unimaginable that Callen would follow in her uncle's footsteps, but she did go to Florida A&M University in Tallahassee, a historically Black college, known at the time as the Florida Agricultural and Mechanical College for Negroes. At that time, nursing was not a college-based education, and so she went to the Georgia Infirmary for her nursing education.

Callen then went as a "nurse missionary" through the Episcopal Church to Berkeley County, South Carolina, for what was to have been a temporary position—and there she remained. She actively worked as a midwife and nurse until her retirement in 1971 and then provided elder care and other community service. Over six decades of practice, it is estimated that Callen attended 600 to 800 births.

Callen arrived in Berkeley County in 1923 and set up what would now be called a midwifery and maternity care service, working out of her own home and traveling on poor roads and often through bad conditions to the homes of birthing women. The area was 98 percent African American and very poorly serviced, without phones, paved roads, electricity, and other basic services for much of her career there.

In 1936, Callen was brought into the public health service of the area and became a public health nurse, expanding her practice to the education of other women in the community as midwives and what we would now call nursing assistants. She not only cared for pregnant and birthing people but also gave vaccinations and provided basic infant and child medical and nursing services. In 1943, Callen went to the Maternity

Center at Tuskegee Institute of Alabama for a six-month course to expand her skills That program is patronizingly described in places such as Wikipedia as "almost as advanced as a doctor's."

Her work became known to a journalist/photographer named Eugene Smith, who had done a photo essay in *LIFE* magazine in 1948 called "Country Doctor" on a white physician in the remote areas of Colorado. *LIFE* published his photo essay on Callen on December 3, 1951, and called it "Nurse Midwife." What we now understand as a nurse-midwife was only just coming into being in the 1940s and 1950s. Callen's role clearly included both nursing and midwifery. Honors came to Callen late in life, beginning with a 1981 award as Outstanding Older South Carolinian. In 1984, she was recipient of the Alexis de Tocqueville Society Award, and in 1989, the year before her death, she was given an honorary degree from the Medical University of South Carolina.

Callen was invited to the White House in the 1980s, under Ronald Reagan, but she felt her ongoing work was more important than leaving for Washington. The quote attributed to her most often is "Let me live in my house by the side of the road and be a friend to man." And by "man" she most clearly also meant women and children.

DeLee, Joseph (1869–1942)

Joseph Bolivar DeLee is often credited as the "father of obstetrics." He was also a staunch opponent of midwifery, contributing to much of the attempted delegitimization of midwives reported in Chapter 1. His very influential article published in the *American Journal of Obstetrics and Gynecology* in 1920 was titled "The Prophylactic Forceps Operation." In it, he urged the prophylactic (intended to prevent disease or harm) use of not only forceps but a host of medications and procedures that became standard in American obstetrics. The procedure he advocated for a routine, normal birth required sedating the people during labor and giving ether for the descent of the fetus. The baby was then removed from the unconscious person with forceps, a pair of tongs that fit around the baby's head and was used to pull the baby out. An incision through the skin and muscle of the perineum, an *episiotomy*, was done before the forceps were applied. The placenta was also removed, and medications were used to prevent postpartum hemorrhage.

DeLee thought that, for the birthing person, birth was comparable to falling on a pitchfork and driving the handle through her perineum, and, for the baby, labor was like having its head crushed in a door. Using these analogies, DeLee was able to conclude that labor was "abnormal": "In both cases, the cause of the damage, the fall on the pitchfork and the crushing of the door, is pathogenic, that is disease-producing, and anything pathogenic is pathologic or abnormal."

As we now understand it, each of these interventions, rather than being prophylactic, are actually the cause of harm and increase the risk of bad outcomes. *Iatrogenic harm* is the term used for medically caused damage, and DeLee's prophylactic use of forceps was the basis of considerable iatrogenic damage. But DeLee's procedures became standard; for example, the first empirical study to determine the long-term effectiveness of episiotomies was not done until the 1970s, and the results indicated that they cause rather than prevent tearing. DeLee claimed that the episiotomy would restore "virginal conditions" to be "better than new." It was not uncommon all through the1970s and 1980s, as partners were permitted into the delivery rooms, to hear obstetricians assuring men that they were sewing their wives up "good and tight."

DeLee is said to have regretted his attempt at prophylaxis.

Friedman, Emanuel (1927–)

Emanuel Friedman, MD, is a professor emerita at Harvard University. He is best known for his influential work on the timing of the stages of labor. He introduced what is known as *Friedman curve*, or what he called a "graphicostatistical analysis of labor," in seven separate articles between 1954 and 1959 in the major *American Journal of Obstetrics*. He observed labors, computed the average length of time they took, broke labor into separate "phases," and found the average length of each phase. He did this separately for primiparas (first births) and for multiparas (people with previous births). He computed the averages and the statistical limits—a measure of the amount of variation. Take the example of height. If we computed heights for people, we could measure many people, get an average, and say how likely it was for someone to be much taller or much shorter than average. A woman over six feet tall is a statistical abnormality. What Friedman did was to make a connection between statistical normality and physiological normality, leading to the medical treatment of statistical abnormality. Using this logic, we could say that a woman of six feet, two inches is not only unusually tall, but that she should be medically treated for her "height condition."

Labors that were statistically abnormally too short did not get treated. Those that were too long, did. The medical treatments are the same as those for the induction of labor: rupture of the membranes, the administration of hormones, and cesarean section. This has become standard obstetrical management and resulted in the average length of labor in hospitals becoming shorter over the years.

These interventions in labors that appear to be a physiologically normal are now being more actively questioned. Generally, midwives will examine the person's experience of labor, and if they are progressing and doing well, without signs of fetal distress, they permit the labor to develop at its own pace.

Gaskin, Ina May (1940–)

Ina May Gaskin is a widely publicized midwife in popular culture. Her 1975 book *Spiritual Midwifery* brought together the counterculture movements of the 1960s and 1970s and the politics of childbirth. It should be noted, however, that midwifery has always had a long and continuous history in the United States, particularly among Black, Indigenous, and people of color (see chapter 1).

Gaskin came to midwifery, as so many contemporary American people, after a badly managed obstetrical birth, in this case involving the unnecessary use of forceps. Some years later, she was part of a caravan following her husband, Steven Gaskin, on a speaking tour; they left San Francisco and eventually settled in a commune known as "the Farm" in Tennessee. People became pregnant and gave birth along that tour, and Ina May Gaskin grew from a supportive helper into the role of midwife. Gaskin eventually established a birth center and midwifery education program at the Farm.

Gaskin was a founder and the first president of the Midwives Alliance of North America (MANA; see MANA entry). She went on to write other books, including guides to childbirth and breastfeeding.

Joseph, Jennie (1959–)

Jennie Joseph is a British Black midwife who was trained in Great Britain. She moved to the United States in 1989, bringing her wide experience of births in European and British hospitals to the American setting. She became a major force in Florida midwifery, serving as the chair of Florida's State Council of Licensed Midwives for many years. She has been active and instrumental in the larger U.S. midwifery world. Her work has drawn attention from such mainstream media sources as Every Mother Counts, CBS, and the *New York Times*.

Joseph observed the high rates of complications in pregnancy among African Americans and began to work to improve outcomes. She opened the Birth Place, a world-renowned birth center, in a suburb of Orlando, Florida, in 1955; it takes any patient, with or without insurance or money, and at any point in pregnancy. Her patients, mostly Black and Latina, are the groups with the highest rates of prematurity and other complications, and yet, at her center, the rate of prematurity is half the local and national averages. Joseph attributes this success to the care and dignity with which each of her clients are treated.

She named her approach to perinatal practice "the JJ Way" and has trademarked that phrase. The core principles are access, connections, knowledge, and empowerment. By *access*, she means that people—as patients or providers—should have access to equitable, evidence-based, quality care and support, including immediate and unrestricted access to services and systems, regardless of their ability to pay. *Connections* refers to the importance of relationships. Her model encourages connections for patient and provider to each other, to the baby, and to the community. *Knowledge* is based on practical and evidence-based ways to improve outcomes and to avoid retraumatizing the patient or the provider. *Empowerment* similarly refers to both patient and provider, allowing them to be heard and to exercise control inside their systems, agencies, and organizations.

The Birth Place is the clinical arm of the larger organization Joseph founded in 1998, Commonsense Childbirth Inc. Commonsense Childbirth provides midwifery education through the Commonsense Childbirth School of Midwifery housed in Florida. The Commonsense Childbirth School of Midwifery is the first and only nationally accredited Black-owned midwifery school. Training and courses are also offered for a variety of provider roles, in addition to midwifery, including lactation educators, community health workers, doulas, childbirth educators, and more.

Commonsense Childbirth is a major actor in building a movement toward Reproductive Justice. The organization is part of the National Perinatal Task Force, whose report issued in March 2018, with Joseph as one of the authors, "Building a

Movement to Birth a More Just and Loving World," provides a detailed analysis of the problems and concerns with American maternity care, especially as it impacts women of color, and specific approaches, including the JJ Way, for making improvements. Jennie Joseph has been instrumental in not only examining but also positively addressing these issues.

Kitzinger, Sheila (1929–2015)

Sheila Kitzinger was an anthropologist who studied childbirth in her own native United Kingdom and around the world, and she was also an activist who promoted a nonmedicalized, woman-centered approach to birth. She lectured widely, in both academic and activist settings, and wrote over twenty books and countless articles and published interviews.

Her first book, *The Experience of Childbirth* (1962), presented her critique of obstetrics as it was practiced at the time: routine separation of the laboring woman from her friends, family and partner; routine episiotomy (the surgical incision to open the vagina); and separation of the baby from the mother immediately after birth, among other issues. Her data-based, woman-centered critique, showing, for example, that episiotomies actually cause more deep tears rather than preventing them, influenced practice first in the United Kingdom and eventually around the world, including the United States.

In her first book, Kitzinger did write about her own experiences of home birth, but she went beyond the personal to bring an anthropologist's eye to the issue. In this, she went beyond what Marjorie Karmel had done in *Thank You, Dr. Lamaze*, the 1959 book that offered the first such widely read feminist's perspective on birth. Kitzinger opened the door for the social scientists who followed, many of whom are cited in this volume, including Nancy Stoller Shaw, Anne Oakley, Barbara Katz Rothman, and Robbie Davis Floyd.

Kitzinger wrote before second-wave feminism but very clearly had a feminist analysis. She saw birth as a psychosexual event, not merely the physical extraction of a fetal parasite from its host, as medicine did and in some ways still does. She understood birth to be a life transition and a site of power, as people struggled to regain control over their own bodies from the medical establishment.

Kitzinger was a key figure in the Childbirth Education Association, an international organization, as well as the National Childbirth Trust in the United Kingdom.

Lawlor, Mary

Mary Lawlor is the executive director of the National Association of Certified Professional Midwives (NACPM). In the mid-1970s, she was invited to a home birth and experienced, as she put it, the "call" to midwifery. In 1975, she moved to Vermont, where she joined a home birth collective, began reading and learning more about midwifery, and eventually began teaching classes herself and attending births as a support person. Lawlor gave birth to her daughter at home in 1976, surrounded by family and friends.

In the early 1980s, Lawlor moved to El Paso for midwifery school and returned to Vermont as a midwife, working with a local physician. She worked independently as a midwife for 15 years in that physician's office, serving many families and supporting the presence of midwifery in the community. Eventually, she opened her own office, and, in 2007, she opened the Monadnock Birth Center, which is still operating today. This birth center was the manifestation of a long dream to make the Midwifery Model of Care visible and accessible in the community.

After the certified professional midwife (CPM) credential was first issued in 1994, Lawlor began working toward the advancement of the credential, first by organizing so that midwives could perform vaginal births after cesarean (VBAC) and eventually participating in a seminal task force meeting in 2001 that gathered to create an organizational home for the credential; thus, the National Association of Certified Professional Midwives (NACPM) was established. Lawlor was a founder of NACPM in 2001 and president of the board for 10 years, and she became the executive director in 2012. She remains a passionate advocate for midwives and for childbearing people's access to the care of midwives, for improving care for all birthing people, and for eliminating racial inequities in midwifery and maternity care and the unconscionable racial disparities in birth outcomes.

Lawlor has participated in, and greatly influenced, the United State Midwifery Education, Regulation, and Association (US MERA), spearheading the design of an active state chapter program and helping to establish two midwife of color positions on the board of directors and two public members. She has worked tirelessly to strengthen the staff of NACPM and the CPM workforce as a whole.

Loftman, Patricia O. (1949–)

Patricia O. Loftman, CNM, LM, MS, FACNM, has been a trailblazing pioneer for contemporary midwives of color, especially at the American College of Nurse-Midwives, where she served as chair of the Midwives of Color Committee, among other positions. She has worked to bring the history of midwifery, especially the history of African American midwifery, into public discourse as well as within the midwifery community itself.

Loftman received a bachelor of science in nursing from Skidmore College and her master of science as a certified nurse-midwife from Columbia University. She provided primary and reproductive health care to women and developed expertise in providing care to women whose pregnancies were complicated by chemical dependency or HIV infection.

Loftman served as a member of the United States Public Health Service Task Force on the Use of Zidovudine to Reduce Perinatal Transmission and was a consultant for developing the first Recommendations for HIV Counseling and Voluntary Testing for Pregnant Women. She participated in discussions related to mandatory testing of pregnant women and partner notification with the Center for Women's Policy Studies as a member of the Planning Workshop of the Office of AIDS Research at the National Institutes of Health. She was also chair of the Women's Health/Clinical Care Group that led to Harlem Hospital Center becoming the first World Health Organization Baby Friendly Hospital in New York City.

Loftman has served as a clinical preceptor for midwifery students, been a national advocate for quality health care for women of color, and continues to promote the midwifery profession through active participation on various American College of Nurse-Midwives (ACNM) task forces and committees. In addition to having served as chair of the American College of Nurse-Midwives, Midwives of Color Committee, she also served as a member of the American College of Nurse-Midwives' board of directors.

Loftman retired in 2010 from Harlem Hospital Center after a midwifery career that spanned 30 years.

Courtesy of Patricia Loftman

Monroe, Shafia

Shafia Monroe founded the International Center for Traditional Childbearing (ICTC) in 1991. The organization focused on the care of pregnant women of color and their families, with a goal of creating more midwives and doulas of color. The ICTC was a foundational organization for Black midwives especially. It organized the International Black Midwives and Healers Conference, which brought midwives together from around the world. In 2018, the ICTC became the National Association to Advance Black Birth (see entry in this chapter).

Monroe learned about midwifery as a young woman and began her journey to becoming a midwife by becoming a nurse's aide at Boston City Hospital when she was 17 years old. What she saw there, working in the postpartum ward, was the poor care, the disrespect, and the unnecessary and harmful interventions that women, and particularly women of color, were subjected to. She became involved locally with the Massachusetts Midwives Alliance, which was training women to become midwives, and reached out globally to find other midwives "who looked like me," women of color and specifically of African descent.

Monroe holds a BA in sociology and a master's in public health, and she has worked as a midwife for much of her career. She worked toward bringing culturally competent care to women and families of color and found that one approach was to bring in doulas. In 2002, she created the ICTC Full Circle Doula Training program to train people in the legacy of the African American midwife. Her training program is aimed at reducing infant and maternal mortality and morbidity and improving the experience of birth for the women and their families by providing more competent care providers. Monroe worked to create a program in Oregon that provided a national model for Medicaid reimbursement for doulas and the first state-based doula-credentialing program.

Monroe's many awards and honors include the Lifetime Achievement Award for Human Right from the Midwives of Alliance of North America; the Dr. Hildrus A. Poindexter Award from the National Black Caucus of Health Workers; the American Public Health Association's Women of Excellence Health and Wellness Award; the Delta Sigma Theta Sorority, Inc., Life Time Achievement Award; the Human Rights in Childbirth's Life Time Achievement Service Award for Community Health; the Midwife Hero Award from the American College of Nurse-Midwives' Midwives of Color Committee; and the Unsung Shero Award, Sista, LLC. She is also featured in the "Women Making History in Portland" mural.

Courtesy of Shafia Monroe

Myers, Suzy (1949–)

In 1971, Suzy Myers began her midwifery career in Seattle when she joined a collective of feminists starting a health clinic. Born in New York City, she had been an activist in high school during the civil rights movement; in college, she protested the Vietnam War; and she arrived in Seattle in her early twenties as the women's movement was emerging seeking meaningful ways to work as a women's health care reform activist. Being a health care practitioner was *not* part of her plan, but that quickly changed as the new Fremont Women's Clinic opened and began training "lay paramedics" to help provide care to low-income women. By 1975, the Fremont Birth Collective had formed to provide home birth services, and Myers was one of those chosen to train as a midwife, with one experienced midwife and two family practice physicians as their teachers. Thus began a 40-year career as a practicing midwife, educator, researcher, and activist.

In 1978, Myers was a cofounder of the Seattle Midwifery School (SMS) and became part of the exciting project of developing one of the first formal education programs of its kind in the United States. At the same time, she and her midwifery partner, Marge Mansfield, grew their successful clinical practice, Seattle Home Maternity Service and Childbirth Center, caring for more than 2,000 families over the next three decades and serving as clinical preceptors to scores of student midwives.

Always drawn to the bigger picture, Myers continued to be involved in support of the development of professional midwifery, locally and nationally. In the 1980s, she was active in legislative reform of Washington's Midwifery Act and helped launch the Midwives' Association of Washington State, and, having understood that maternity care reform is a public health issue, in 1988, she earned a master's degree in public health from the University of Washington.

In 2009, as she retired from active clinical practice, Myers helped lead SMS in an intentional merger with Bastyr University to create the Department of Midwifery there, the first regionally accredited, direct-entry program in the United States to grant a master's degree in midwifery, and she became its first department chair, a position she held until her retirement in 2018.

A defining theme in Myers's life's work has been the urgent need to improve maternity care that had been made clear by examining the relatively poor pregnancy and birth outcomes in the United States and especially how systemic racism contributes to disparate outcomes for Black and brown families. Her national work on the board of directors of the National Association of Certified Professional Midwives (NACPM) from 2002 to 2013 provided an invaluable experience in working for integration of midwifery care nationally, influencing health care policy, and deepening her understanding of the imperative to address racism, including within the ranks of the midwifery profession. Although retired, Myers continues her advocacy work, which is especially focused on supporting Black and other people of color to become midwives and serve communities so desperately in need of them.

Courtesy of Suzy Myers

Sanger, Margaret (1879–1966)

Margaret Sanger is a controversial historical figure. She was born into a poor family, 1 of 11 surviving children. Her mother died of tuberculosis. Sanger went on to become a nurse and worked in New York City, providing care to poor families living in tenement housing. Sanger saw that people in poverty were having repeated pregnancies that they did not want but had no way to prevent. While wealthier people had access to some forms of contraception and to relatively safe, if illegal, abortions, poor women had none of that. Sanger saw that when people were pregnant and could not afford to care for the children they already had, they took great risks with illegal and unsafe abortions. Too many pregnancies, whether resulting in many live births or repeated abortions, presented risks to the health and lives of these people. In 1916, she opened up the first birth control clinic in the United States in Brooklyn, New York.

Sanger began teaching and writing about how to prevent unwanted pregnancies, popularizing the term "birth control." At that time, it was illegal in the United States to even write about sexuality: The Comstock Act of 1873 was a federal statute that made it a criminal offense to import, mail, or transport in interstate commerce any "obscene literature" or any information or objects for the prevention of conception. In 1914, she launched a newsletter "The Woman Rebel," which promoted birth control. She also prepared a 16-page pamphlet called "Family Limitation," further educating people about preventing pregnancies. In her work and its distribution, in her commitment to access to information about birth control as a free speech issue, Sanger put herself in violation of federal law. She was repeatedly arrested and was indicted for violating postal obscenity laws. The resulting trial and appeal received considerable news coverage, and the conversation on contraception reached the mainstream.

Sanger organized the American Birth Control League in 1921, which later became known as Planned Parenthood, and served as its president until 1928. She organized a World Population Conference in Geneva in 1927 and an International Conference for Doctors and Scientists in 1930. Bringing the medical field into the discussion was invaluable: the Medical Research Bureau, headed by Dr. Helen Stone, began the first organized birth control research, and in 1936, birth control under medical direction became legal when the Comstock Act was struck down.

Sanger worked to bring birth control to people in the United States but throughout the world. She was involved with progressive labor movements and with early feminist groups such as the European Free Love Movement, which argued against the double standard in which men were understood to have sexual needs and interests but women were not.

Sanger, however, was a eugenicist and promoted ideas of selective reproduction. In 2020, the Planned Parenthood of Greater New York announced its intent to remove Sanger's name from its Manhattan Health Center following a commitment to become an anti-racist organization.

Sims, J. Marion (1813–1883)

James Marion Sims is a problematic historical figure who has been called the "father of modern gynecology." He was a physician, who was born, raised, and educated in the South during slavery. He became interested in the condition known as "vaginal fistulas," tears between the vagina and the bladder, rectum, and other tissues. These tears were most commonly caused by obstructed births. They were painful and resulted in incontinence, the leaking of urine or fecal matter. Sims developed techniques and tools to address such issues.

However, Sims developed his techniques by practicing and experimenting on enslaved women, some of whom he returned to their owners and at least one of whom he bought specifically to work on (see chapter 1). Although ether for anesthesia came into use early on in his years of developing the surgical repair, he chose not to use it. There was a racist medical argument that ether was too difficult and risky, and there was a specific argument that Black people feel less pain than white people.

Drugs and other procedures in gynecology and in medicine at large have too often been developed on poor people, people of color, and people in underresourced countries, and when considered perfected enough for use, they were then brought to wealthier white people.

In 2018, Sims's New York City statue was removed from Central Park.

Smith, Margaret Charles (1906–2004)

Margaret Charles Smith, a licensed African American midwife originally from Eutaw, Alabama, who practiced for decades in Greene County, Alabama, is one of the most recognized midwives in the United States. While countless African American midwives cared for mothers, Black and white, from the time of enslavement until their practices were eliminated in 1981, Smith was the first to tell her story as coauthor of a book, *Listen to Me Good: The Life Story of an Alabama Midwife* (Ohio State University Press, 1996).

With only a few years of formal elementary school education, Smith provided care that resulted in healthy birthing outcomes for thousands of mothers and babies. White supremacist ideology and Jim Crow segregation denied most African American women access to the medical services and hospitals in the Deep South, thus providing a space for the skills and strengths of traditional African American midwifery care to flourish.

Licensed to practice as a midwife in 1949, Smith integrated wisdom from her enslaved grandmother about plant medicine and culturally based birthing customs with lessons learned from an apprenticeship with an experienced African American midwife who she followed and assisted for a year. Later, Smith traveled to Tuskegee Institute, where she enrolled in a weeklong training workshop for lay midwives at Andrew Memorial Hospital. Smith also assisted nurses at the Greene County Health Department's maternity clinic housed in a small isolated cabin that women seeking care from a midwife were required to attend at least twice. Although often caring for mothers in impoverished circumstances without electricity or running water, Smith's holistic midwifery care contributed to positive outcomes in the overwhelming majority of the cases she attended.

When Alabama made it illegal for lay midwives to practice in 1981, Smith began capturing local and national attention as a historic African American midwife who advocated for continuing the practices of lay midwives like herself. In 1983,

Smith was the first Black person to receive the key to the city of Eutaw. Two year later, the Black Women's Health Project honored Smith at Spelman College. In the years that followed, the Boston Women's Health Book Collective, the Midwives Alliance of North America, and the American College of Nurse-Midwives were among the diverse groups that recognized Smith. In 2003, a year before her death at the age of 98, Smith traveled to Washington, DC, where she was honored by the Congressional Black Caucus. Inducted posthumously into the Alabama Women's Hall of Fame in 2011, Smith now stands alongside Helen Keller, Coretta Scott King, Rosa Parks, and other legendary Alabama women because of her historic contributions as a midwife and advocate for women.

Courtesy of Linda Janet Holmes

Stoney, George C. (1916–2012)

George C. Stoney was a documentary filmmaker who had a long and influential career and became known as the "father of public access television." As a young man, Stoney had observed the presence of the Black midwives in his native South and was interested in doing a documentary but had no access. He worked with the Georgia Department of Public Health to create a "training film." The resulting documentary, *All My Babies: A Midwife's Own Story*, produced in 1953, was his first major film.

In the 1950s, before what became known as the civil rights movement, there was a space in white American culture for a kind of romanticism about rural life. Without acknowledging the poverty, let alone the causes of that poverty, the lives of "simpler people" in "simpler times" was romanticized. The postwar United States was dealing with increasing industrialization, with more and more premade manufactured and standardized food and clothing, and a domestic life that had turned to consumption. Rural life in general, and perhaps Black rural life in particular, came to be seen in its contrast, but not entirely as a negative contrast.

With regard to birth and midwifery, this can be seen through the eyes of two white men who made contributions in publicizing African American midwifery. Eugene Smith did a photo essay on Maude Callen, a Black woman trained as a professional nurse who was working as a midwife and essentially as a primary care provider in a deeply poor Black community in South Carolina. His work was published in *LIFE* magazine, where he had earlier profiled a white man physician practicing in a white rural area of Colorado (see the Maude E. Callen entry).

Stoney's 1953 film, perhaps especially when seen through a contemporary eye, makes apparent the implicit racism and medical domination of the time. In one scene, a room full of Black midwives, including the central character of the film, the midwife Mary Francis Hill Coley, who had attended over 3,000 births in her career, are being taught how to tie a knot by a white nurse. The nurse is "training" people like Coley on how to literally tie a knot for cutting off the umbilical cord; they practice on string as she checks their work. In another scene, a white physician lectures these midwives on the importance of cleanliness in preventing infection, with a haunting image later in the film of Coley waking in the night to clean her equipment. It is well known that infections are far more likely and dangerous in hospital settings than at home, and Stoney had noted the care and cleanliness Coley used; however, the image the medical authorities who wanted the film for training purposes put forward is that the "dirty" midwives are the source of infection. The film also shows the midwife turning the birthing person in their own bed, from the more physiological and culturally normative side-lying position for birth to the medically approved on-your-back, knees-up variation on the lithotomy position. These are among the medically approved "training" aspects of the film, which was funded and approved for the training of community midwives.

Through Stoney's work, this hidden-from-white-society role of Black midwives entered public consciousness. Coley became known a "towering figure" of the American documentary tradition. The film came to be shown in a variety of contexts, far beyond what the Department of Health ever imagined. It is an introduction to home birth and midwifery for those who might never otherwise have heard of that tradition.

Barbara Katz Rothman, in one of the first sociological studies of birth in the United States, credits seeing the film in a college health education course—contrasted with a French Lamaze film shown the same session—as setting her on the path to a home birth. The attentive gentle care, the respect shown the birthing women, the midwife at her home, and the family at hand contrasted powerfully with a person lying flat on their back, knees up, on a delivery table with attendants telling her how to breathe in rhythm.

The film was chosen as a "cultural, historically and artistically significant work" and placed in the National Film Registry by the Library of Congress in 2002. George Stoney went on to produce many other important films. He founded his own production company and worked in public television to allow community voices to be heard. He was also a professor at the New York University Tisch School of the Arts.

Social Scientists Studying Birth

There are now many social scientists who study issues related to pregnancy and birth, and in the United States, that has not always been the case. It was only as women moved into the social sciences that birth became recognized as an area of interest and study. In this section, we highlight profiles of some of these trailblazers, social scientists who saw birth as an important issue that was well worth their intellectual attention.

Davis-Floyd, Robbie (1951–), Anthropologist

Dr. Robbie Davis-Floyd's work has played a significant role in connecting the midwifery community with the academic world and anthropology in particular. Her first book, *Birth as an American Rite of Passage* (University of California Press,

1992), focused on the role that industrialization played in the medical management of birth. This goes beyond the medical understanding of the body as a machine to be technologically managed and includes the hospital as a factory-like industrial setting.

Davis-Floyd went on to work on the expanded and seriously updated 1993 version of Brigitte Jordan's *Birth in Four Cultures*, bringing that book back into print. She has more recently served as a coeditor of a greatly expanded anthropological analysis of birth in different cultures, *Birth in Eight Cultures* (coedited with Melissa Cheyney, Waveland Press, 2019), which focuses on the contestations around birth in Brazil, Greece, Japan, Mexico, the Netherlands, New Zealand, Tanzania, and the United States.

Davis-Floyd has consistently addressed the "cultural battle" that birth is in the United States and around the world, cowriting and coediting with social scientists and birth activists. She remains active in the field and is a senior research fellow at the University of Texas, Austin.

Jordan, Brigitte (1938–2016), Anthropologist

Although Margaret Mead and other women anthropologists had of course paid some attention to childbirth practices in different cultures, it was not until Dr. Brigitte Jordan published *Birth in Four Cultures: A Crosscultural Investigation of Childbirth in Yucatan, Holland, Sweden, and the United States* in 1978 that specific attention was paid by anthropology to American childbirth practices. The book has been reprinted with additional material many times, including a fourth edition that was revised and expanded by Robbie Davis-Floyd.

The original research for the first edition was begun in the 1970s and was originally written as a dissertation in 1975. Over the years since, more original research has been added, including systematic videotaping of the birth process in each of the cultures studied. What Jordan found was how very deeply interconnected the physical experience of birth and the cultural expectations are. What a labor looks, sounds, and feels like is shaped by the cultural and social norms.

Jordan observed the extreme medicalization of childbirth in both Sweden and the United States, with almost all births occurring under medical management in hospital settings. While there was some discussion of "natural" childbirth in the United States, which had grown considerably in the years following her original research, she found that American childbirth had become more polarized, with a dramatic increase in surgery and technologization, as evidenced by the ever-rising cesarean section rate and the increasingly ubiquitous use of fetal monitoring on the one hand and the vocal and politicized movement that advocated a return to a more physiological way of birthing, on the other. In Sweden, in contrast to the United States, she found a strong consensus about the management of birth, with both providers and birthing people expecting increased pharmacologization and technologization of birth. Swedish birthing people are involved in choices about which medications, sedations, and anesthesia are used, but they were not, as American birthing people increasingly were, rejecting medical management.

In Holland, or the Netherlands as it is named, birth that is natural, physiological, and managed with a minimum of interference continued to be valued; midwives attended most births; and at the time of Jordan's original research, more than half of all births took place at home. This number has been dropping over the years since. In the Yucatan, she found a strong and viable "ethno-obstetrics," an attempt to not only train traditional midwives in the direction of modern medicine but also to work with physicians to understand traditional birth practices.

The anthropology of birth was greatly informed by Jordan's book and continues to build on her work. She died in 2016.

Raphael, Dana (1926–2016), Anthropologist

In her scholarship, Dr. Dana Raphael observed how breast-feeding was handled in different cultures. She saw that in cultures in which people were helped, tended to, and taken care of, breastfeeding went well. This was in strong contrast to the American model she observed around her: people were left very much to their own devices, in their own homes, with no help with childcare for their other children and no release from their household and other obligations.

Raphael emphasized the role of helper(s). As she thought of this, "mothering the mother," a Greek woman suggested the word *doula* to describe that position. Doula means "maidservant," but Raphael used the word in a more respectful way. She noted that most cultures provide some of that kind of care, someone who is usually but not always a woman, who is usually but not always experienced in mothering, breastfeeding, and other work. The key part of the role as Raphael used it was the focus on the mother, someone whose role and job it was to take care of the mother so that she could take care of the baby.

The term *doula* was used in Raphael's 1966 dissertation and then brought into a more public realm with the publication of her 1976 book, *The Tender Gift: Breastfeeding*. In the decades since, the use of the term has expanded from its original postpartum focus to include doulas for pregnancy care and in particular for the birth, someone who is brought in specifically to provide caring attention to the birthing person.

Raphael, along with Margaret Mead, founded the Human Lactation Center in 1975, and she continued her work and her advocacy in support of people in their role as mother.

Roberts, Dorothy (1956–), Sociologist and Law Scholar

Dr. Dorothy Roberts's scholarship has influenced many academics, activists, and birth workers in the United States. Her pathbreaking work in law and public policy focuses on urgent contemporary issues in health, Reproductive Justice, social justice, and bioethics, especially as they impact the lives of women, children, and African Americans. Her major books include *Fatal Invention: How Science, Politics, and Big Business Re-Create Race in the Twenty-First Century* (New Press, 2011); *Shattered Bonds: The Color of Child Welfare* (Basic Books, 2002); and *Killing the Black Body: Race, Reproduction, and the Meaning of Liberty* (Pantheon, 1997). She is the author of more than 100 scholarly articles and book chapters and is a coeditor of six books on such topics as constitutional law and women and the law.

Roberts is the University of Pennsylvania's 14th Penn Integrates Knowledge Professor with joint appointments in the Departments of Africana Studies and Sociology and the Law School, where she holds the inaugural Raymond Pace and Sadie Tanner Mossell Alexander chair. She is also founding director of the Penn Program on Race, Science & Society in the Center for Africana Studies.

Roberts serves on the board of directors of the American Academy of Political and Social Science, and her work has been supported by the American Council of Learned Societies, the National Science Foundation, the Robert Wood Johnson Foundation, the Harvard Program on Ethics & the Professions, and the Stanford Center for the Comparative Studies in Race & Ethnicity. Recent recognitions of her work include election to the National Academy of Medicine in 2017, the Society of Family Planning's 2016 Lifetime Achievement Award, and the American Psychiatric Association's 2015 Solomon Carter Fuller Award.

Roberts, Lynn, Public Health Scholar

Dr. Lynn Roberts is a public health scholar and activist. Her work examines the intersections of race, gender, and other marginalities in adolescent dating relationships, juvenile justice, and reproductive health policies as well as the impact of models of collaborative inquiry and teaching on civic and political engagement.

The City University of New York (CUNY) has been Roberts's academic home since 1995. Prior to joining CUNY, she oversaw the development, implementation, and evaluation of several prevention programs for women and youth in New York City. She has also served on the board of SisterSong Women of Color Reproductive Justice Collective and coedited an anthology on Reproductive Justice (CUNY Feminist Press, 2017). Since 2015, she has been a consultant to the New York City Department of Health and Mental Hygiene in support of their efforts to integrate a sexual and Reproductive Justice framework in their work. She also serves as a collaborator for the Black Mamas Matter Alliance.

Rothman, Barbara Katz (1948–), Sociologist

While Nancy Stoller Shaw was the first sociologist to seriously address childbirth in America, Dr. Barbara Katz Rothman was the first sociologist to look at the developing midwifery movement, an attempt to resolve the concerns Stoller Shaw addressed by moving birth out of medical management and into midwifery care and the home. Her book *In Labor: Women and Power in the Birthplace* was based on in-depth interviews and ethnographic work with midwives in the New York City metropolitan area who were attending births at home. Some had been trained in other countries where home birth was available; most were American nurse-midwives who had never seen a nonmedicalized birth. They found, doing home births, that birth was not what they had been trained to see. Rothman's research began in the mid 1970s and resulted in the publication *In Labor* in 1979.

What Rothman found was that the midwives were not just being "kinder," "gentler," and more caring in their care, but they came to have a fundamentally different understanding of what was happening in childbirth. Rather than seeing a fetal patient in need of extraction from a maternal barrier, as the obstetricians spoke, these midwives were seeing a person who was actively engaged in labor and birth, not "being delivered" but "giving birth." Rothman named these two different understandings the "medical model" and the "midwifery model." The term *Midwives Model of Care* has since entered the lexicon of midwifery.

The medical model sees the body as essentially a machine, with the male body taken as a norm. Pregnancy and birth are at best complications, stresses on the system; at worst, they are disease-like states. In either case, pregnancy and birth need treatment and medical management. The midwifery model was person-centered, and birth was viewed as an organic, mind-body experience, a physiological accomplishment rather than a problem to be solved technologically.

Rothman went on to publish other books related to pregnancy and childbirth, including *The Tentative Pregnancy*, the first sociological study of women's experiences of prenatal screening and selective abortion, and a recent book comparing the food movement and its fight against industrialization with the birth movement, *A Bun in the Oven: How the Food and Birth Movements Resist Industrialization*. She is also coeditor of this volume.

Stoller Shaw, Nancy (1942–), Sociologist

Dr. Nancy Stoller Shaw (also now known as Nancy Stoller) wrote the first book-length, sociological analysis of childbirth in the United States in her book *Forced Labor: Maternity Care in the United States*, published by Pergamon Studies in Critical Sociology on January 1, 1974. Starting in 1967, she spent over three years doing participant observation and ethnographic research at a maternity care hospital in the United States using the principles of "grounded theory," following in the tradition of other classic sociological studies of medical institutions. The work was quite critical of the way that childbirth was managed in this setting, as indicated in its title.

Stoller Shaw identified five factors that decreased patient control and dehumanization: (1) the medical monopoly on childbirth care, driving out the midwives and midwifery care; (2) the hospital setting itself, which required standardization and the inherent degradation of the patient as a work object, cut off from all family and friends; (3) the specialization and fragmentation of care, including the separation of the person under the care of the obstetrician and the baby under the care of the pediatrician, but more generally a lack of personal connection for the birthing person in the system; (4) a reliance on technology, which essentially denied freedom, requiring the birthing person to be a passive recipient of assorted services and drugs rather than an active participant while laboring and birthing the baby; and (5) the use of power and status, in which physicians were higher status than patients in general and female-identifying patients in particular. This unequal distribution of power made it harder for those in power to identify with the people they were ostensibly caring for.

Stoller Shaw was a professor at the University of California, Santa Cruz. When she came up for tenure, she was denied. Her work was not considered "valuable" or sociological enough. She claimed sex discrimination and fought back. Feminist academics around the country rallied, as did the women faculty and staff on her own campus. She ultimately won the case, received the pay she had been owed, and was promoted. She continued her career at the university, becoming chair of community studies, and is now professor emerita.

Organizations

American College of Nurse-Midwives

The American College of Nurse-Midwives, founded in 1955, is the largest professional membership organization of certified nurse-midwives (CNMs) and certified midwives (CMs). To date, there are approximately 13,004 CNMs and 117 CMs practicing in the United States. ACNM seeks to advance the profession by advocating for CNMS and CMs at all levels of government; promoting the development, dissemination, and implementation of quality research, including the bimonthly publication of the *Journal of Midwifery and Women's Health*; supporting midwifery education; and, issuing evidence-based practice recommendations and policy briefs. The Black Midwives Caucus for Reproductive Justice and Birth Equity and the Midwives of Color Committee within ACNM work to building community among midwifery students and currently practicing midwives, and support the development of a representee midwifery workforce. ACNM is a member of the United States Midwifery Education, Regulation, and Association (US MERA) and the International Confederation of Midwives (ICM).

American College of Obstetricians and Gynecologists

The American College of Obstetricians and Gynecologists (ACOG) is the largest professional membership organization of obstetricians and gynecologists (OB-GYN). Founded in 1951, ACOG seeks to advance the profession by producing practice guidelines for providers and educational materials for patients; providing practice management and career support; facilitating programs and initiatives aimed at improving women's health; and, advocating on behalf of members and patients. It publishes the journal *Obstetrics & Gynecology*, known as the "Green Journal," every month.

American Public Health Association

Founded in 1872, The American Public Health Association (APHA) is the only organization that combines a nearly 150-year perspective, a broad-based member community and the ability to influence federal policy to improve the public's health. The COVID-19 global pandemic has shown light on the imperative need for a national public health strategy, for which APHA has always been working toward. APHA has been profoundly influential and is consistently educating the public on why racism along with police violence are public health issues. APHA publishes monthly issues of *American Journal of Public Health*. We wish to draw specific attention to Sexual and Reproductive Health Section (formerly the Population, Reproductive, and Sexual Health Section) of APHA. Founded in 1975, this Section works to improve the health of adults and children by ensuring that sexual and reproductive health remain major domestic and international priorities.

Black Mamas Matter Alliance

The Black Mamas Matter Alliance is a cross-sectoral alliance led by Black women. It centers Black mamas to advocate, drive research, build power, and shift culture for Black perinatal and reproductive health, rights, and justice. The Black Mamas Matter Alliance was sparked by a partnership project between the Center for Reproductive Rights (CRR) and SisterSong Women of Color Reproductive Justice Collective (SisterSong) that began in 2013. The two organizations collaborated on story collection on the obstacles that Southern Black women face in accessing maternal health care, leading to poor maternal health outcomes and persistent racial disparities. These findings were included in a joint report (also written with the National Latina Institute for Reproductive Health), *Reproductive Injustice: Gender and Racial Discrimination in U.S. Health Care*, submitted to the United Nations Committee on the Elimination of Racial Discrimination (CERD).

Monica Simpson of SisterSong, Katrina Anderson of CRR, and Elizabeth Dawes Gay co-organized a convention in Atlanta in June 2015 that brought together experts, activists, and stakeholders from a variety of sectors who were concerned about

Black maternal health. Black Mamas Matter (BMM) was an outcome of this meeting, along with a call to action to produce toolkits for activists in the South working to improve maternal health. Over the course of the next year, CRR, in collaboration with members of BMM, created the Black Mamas Matter Toolkit.

A second convention was held in Atlanta in June 2016 to launch the toolkit and discuss how to implement it in Georgia, where some political momentum on this issue seemed to exist. At this meeting, members identified the myriad strategies needed to effectively tackle the crisis of maternal health (advocacy, culture shift, research, and service provision) and called for a Black women–led initiative to leverage these strategies.

Recognizing the need for the BMM project to become its own entity, CRR and SisterSong initiated a process to create a steering committee to guide BMM into its next phase. In November 2016, BMM hosted its first steering committee retreat. At this two-day meeting, the group decided on the "alliance" structure and crafted a vision, mission, values, goals, and work plan for the upcoming year. Their goals are to change policy, cultivate research, advance care for Black mamas, and shift culture.

To date, the alliance includes close to 30 groups and organizations; a list can be found at https://blackmamasmatter.org /our-members/. The authors especially encourage readers to note the work of Ancient Song Doula Services (NY), Mamatoto Village (DC), National Birth Equity Collaborative (LA), National Black Midwives Alliance (GA), Shafia Monroe Birthing Change (OR), SisterSong Women of Color Reproductive Justice Collective (GA), and Southern Birth Justice Network (FL).

Black Women's Health Imperative

In 1983, Byllye Y. Avery convened a conference at Spelman College, one of the historically Black colleges, in Atlanta, Georgia. Avery was on the board of the National Women's Health Network. She had previously been involved in the founding and running of services focused on abortion access and a birth center. She began a two-year project focused on the health of Black women and convened the conference at Spelman, which was the Black Women's Health Project.

In 1990, the project opened an office in Washington, DC, focused on public policy and education and relocated its central office to the capital in 1995. A rich range of national and local organizations were affiliated with that office, and in 2002, the organization changed its name to the Black Women's Health Imperative and dedicated itself to national programs in health policy, education, research, knowledge, and leadership development to improve the health and save the lives of Black women in the United States.

On its web page, the organization describes its milestones, or achievements, by the decade (https://bwhi.org/our-story/). In its founding decade of 1981–1991, these included convening that first national conference in 1983, the first dedicated specifically to the health concerns of Black women; establishing a center for women's wellness within public housing communities; sending a delegation to Kenya for the United Nations Decade for Women; and publishing a health news magazine called *Vital Signs*. Accomplishments of the second decade, 1992–2002, included more international work, such as participating in an exchange program with women in South Africa; more publications, including "Our Bodies, Our Voices: A Black Women's Primer on Reproductive Health and Rights"; producing videos; and launching the website www.BlackWomensHealth.Org. In the third decade, meetings and publications continued, and the awards began to grow: the 2012 Women's Empowerment Award, grants to conduct wellness programs in five cities, and the 2013 NAACP Literary Image Award. The website www .BlackWomensHealth.org was also named the #1 Resource for Black Women by *Essence* magazine.

The work continues and addresses health concerns of a wide variety: diabetes, reproductive issues, HIV prevention for cis- and transgender women, and more. The organization also continues its work in developing leadership among Black women, in particular through a program My Sisters Keeper for women at historically Black colleges and universities and its focus on policy development.

Elephant Circle

Inspired by elephants who give birth within a circle of support, Elephant Circle envisions a world where all people have a circle of support for the entire perinatal period.

Founded in 2009, Elephant Circle provides expertise and support to individuals and groups on the HOW and WHAT of birth justice which seeks to dismantle systems of oppression for the liberation of all peoples. Founded in 2009, Elephant Circle provides expertise in this area and offers individual and group coaching and consulting, along with Reproductive Justice curriculum development. Indra Lusero, who has contributed an essay in Chapter 3, is the founder and director of Elephant Circle.

In Our Own Voice

In Our Own Voice is a collaboration of organizations concerned with issues of Reproductive Justice for Black women. It was founded by Marcela Howell.

In 1994, a group of Black women gathered in Chicago. They were concerned with the ways that both globally and in the United States the needs of Black women in issues of procreation were not being met. The privacy-based pro-choice movement in particular was of limited value for women of color, as they had minimal access to choice and the means to achieve it. Having participated in the International Conference on Population and Development in Cairo and a variety of national and local conferences in the United States, these Black women came together and launched a new Reproductive Justice movement, focusing specifically on the unmet needs of Black women. They adopted a human rights framework, approaching issues the reproductive rights movement had addressed in a broader social justice context.

Over the years, the language of Reproductive Justice has become more widely used and understood as focusing on the unmet needs of women of color and women in poverty for help and care in all issues of procreation. SisterSong, based in the South of the United States, is perhaps the largest and best known of the Reproductive Justice movements; it was established in 1997 by organizations of women of color, including African American, Native American, Latina, and Asian American women. The membership includes the women it represents and their allies. SisterSong defines *Reproductive Justice* "as the human right to maintain personal bodily autonomy, have children, not have children, and parent the children we have in safe and sustainable communities."

Reproductive Justice thus requires significant social change. Bringing the various organizations together is part of the long-term change strategy to create the societal structures and values to create a world in which Reproductive Justice is to be achieved. Successes have been achieved at some state and local levels, some social awareness has been raised, and the ideas behind the Reproductive Justice movement are in some ways entering into mainstream consciousness.

In Our Own Voice has launched an agenda, "In Our Own Voice: National Black Women's Reproductive Justice Agenda," with abortion rights and access, contraceptive equity, and comprehensive sex education as its key policy issues. Working with Marcela Howell, an advocate, In Our Own Voice has been seeking foundation funding, with increasing success, to create an infrastructure of Black women–centered reproductive and health organizations.

A key principle of the Reproductive Justice approach embodied in In Our Own Voice and other Reproductive Justice organizations is the idea to "Trust Black Women." As all feminist reproductive movements have argued, people have rights of bodily autonomy. A system of services that does not enable people to make their own decisions in their own ways fails them. Black women in particular have not been treated as competent or trustworthy decision makers, most especially in their role as mothers—or in their decision to not become mothers. The legal language of the *Roe* decision allowing access to abortion placed that decision in the hands of "a woman and her doctor." That is not acceptable. In birth, in parenting, in sexuality, in contraception, *all* people need the resources and support to act in their own best interests and to make choices and have access to choices that enable their autonomy.

La Leche League

On a July day in 1956, two mothers at a Christian family movement picnic in Franklin Park, Illinois, sat under a tree and nursed their babies. Throughout the afternoon, mothers walked over to them and said, "I had so wanted to nurse my baby, but . . .." "That's when it really hit us that the problems we had in trying to nurse our babies were common to a lot of mothers," Marion Thompson recalled; it was not any particular person's rare problem but something systemic. That kind of mental leap, made between one's personal problems and a common situation, has variously been called the sociological imagination and consciousness raising. Those two women, along with five others, took that idea and joined together in what eventually became La Leche League International, with thousands of groups in the United States as well as groups in 89 other countries.

By the 1950s, Americans were at least a full generation removed from midwifery and home birth. Standard medical management separated the birthing person and baby at birth for 24 hours of "observation" and then only permitted people to see their babies for brief periods every four hours, but only during daytime shifts. This made breastfeeding very difficult. Babies were given bottles in the hospital, and people did not learn how to put the baby to breast. Physicians wrote out a "formula" (what would ordinarily be called a "recipe" but when written on a prescription pad became known as "formula") for a mix of evaporated milk, corn syrup, and water, with the percentages varying with the age of the baby.

La Leche League argued not only for the superiority of breast milk as the naturally appropriate food for babies but also for encouraging people to trust themselves, to come to know their bodies and their babies, and to learn from what other people experienced with breastfeeding, chestfeeding and baby care rather than entirely rely on the knowledge of the mostly male physicians who had never actually done any of the work of infant and baby care.

La Leche League offers help to anyone dealing with breastfeeding and chestfeeding challenges. Originally, they held group meetings and provided telephone counseling; moving on with the times, they now also hold virtual meetings. La Leche League International leaders are volunteers who have breastfed and are accredited as having been specially trained to provide breastfeeding and chestfeeding help and keeping up to date on medical and other research on breastfeeding.

In the 1980s, La Leche League International was granted the status of consultant with the United Nations Children's Fund (UNICEF) and began to provide certification for lactation consultants.

The name "La Leche League" comes from the Spanish word *leche*, for "milk," and was inspired by a shrine in St. Augustine, Florida, dedicated to "Nuestra Señora de la Leche y Buen Parto" ("Our Lady of Happy Birth and Plentiful Milk").

March for Moms

Founded in 2017, March for Moms aligns the diverse voices of families, health care providers, policymakers, and partners to advocate for mother's and families' health, well-being, and equal access to care. Each year, they hold a march on the National Mall in Washington, D.C. to bring together the diverse voices of everyone who supports the health and well-being of all mothers and their families. They are a repository of state and federal perinatal health data to equip people to advocate to their legislators for systemic change. They encourage people-birthing people and partners and/or family members to share their birth stories to raise awareness about the experiences of people birthing in the United States.

March of Dimes

The idea of a charity specifically focused on one disease, such as breast cancer or Alzheimer's, is now quite commonplace. However, that was not true in 1938 when President Franklin Delano Roosevelt (FDR) founded the National Foundation for Infantile Paralysis, a disease now better known as "polio." Polio is a contagious disease caused by a virus that is easily transmitted through food and water and widely spread in summertime. It was predominantly a childhood disease. Survivors generally experienced some level of permanent paralysis, including those who could no longer breathe and were placed in "iron lungs," living their entire lives in that machine. Roosevelt was 39 when he had polio, and he lost the use of his legs.

At that point in the United States, there was enormous stigma toward any physical disability, and wheelchair users were disparagingly called "crippled" and largely kept out of public life. The curb cuts, wheelchair access, and other accommodations that disability activists worked so hard to achieve, and with which we are now familiar, were not available. Roosevelt went to great trouble to keep his disability out of the public eye, and there are very few images of him in a wheelchair or his being assisted in any way. He is usually shown behind a desk.

FDR founded the organization to enable a quick response to areas experiencing polio epidemics, to provide services to the people in need, and eventually to do research toward prevention and a cure. That ultimately brought funding to Jonas Salk, a young physician who developed a safe and effective vaccine and essentially eliminated polio.

At a public appeal in 1938, the singer Eddie Cantor jokingly asked people to send dimes to the White House to fund the National Foundation for Infantile Paralysis, and people responded quite literally, sending close to $3,000 worth of dimes plus other contributions. The grassroots nature of the organization, funded by the people, is commemorated in its change of name to the March of Dimes. FDR's image was also added to the obverse of the dime in 1946.

Once polio was cured, this well-established, well-funded, and well-run organization turned its attention to other causes of disease and disability, particularly in children and babies. Dr. Virginia Apgar (see entry) became involved, and the switch was to congenital disabilities, including those caused by poor health of the gestational parent, often related to race and poverty in the United States, which is a cause of premature birth. Prematurity is one of the greatest causes of poor infant health. The March of Dimes worked to establish more prenatal care programs and make services available to all pregnant people.

Other work has been more controversial, such as addressing prenatal screening for genetic disorders that cannot be cured and so may result in selective abortion. The March of Dimes currently focuses its mission on the prevention of prematurity, pointing out that it is the number one killer of babies in the United States. From its original work on polio to its current attention to prematurity, the March of Dimes has focused on researching the problems that threaten our children and finding ways to prevent them.

Midwives Alliance of North America

The Midwives Alliance of North America (MANA) was founded in 1982 in response to the growing number of midwives developing out of the emerging home birth movement. MANA brought all kinds of midwives—the certified nurse-midwives (CNMs) and what were then called "lay" midwives—together to develop a new philosophy and mechanisms for direct-entry midwifery. These midwives were not "lay," which is to say untrained and unprofessional; rather, they were being trained and educated in new ways. MANA developed to recognize the evolving nature of midwifery as a profession, cutting across educational pathways.

These midwives came together to establish a nonprofit organization that would be a collective home for all kinds of midwives, recognizing the diversity of paths into midwifery and the shared Midwives Model of Care the organization and its members valued. In April 1982, over a hundred midwives gathered together in Lexington, Kentucky, and began the organization, choosing the name MANA to emphasize the alliance and the mutual support and respect among midwives of different backgrounds and to include the similarly struggling development of midwifery in Canada as in the United States. Among the founders of MANA was Ina May Gaskin (see entry), who became the first president of the organization.

MANA declares itself uniquely positioned to unite and strengthen all midwives through dedication to innovative education, professional development, and recognized autonomous practice. MANA is a member of the United States Midwifery Education, Regulation, and Association (US MERA) and the International Confederation of Midwives (ICM).

National Advocates for Pregnant Women

The National Advocates for Pregnant Women (NAPW) is a nonprofit organization founded by its current executive director, Lynn Paltrow, to protect the rights of pregnant women. While much of American attention to pregnancy rights is focused on access to abortion, Lynn Paltrow works on other cases as a lawyer defending the human rights of pregnant women to control their own bodies and lives.

An early and key case was that of Angela Carder, a 27-year-old woman who had survived a recurrent childhood cancer and became pregnant. In 1987, in her 25th week of pregnancy, the cancer returned. While she, her husband, her family, and her obstetric team focused on providing the best care for Carder, the hospital administrators decided it was appropriate to do a cesarean section and attempt to care for the very premature fetus. They convened a court hearing at the hospital, and against the intention of Carder and her family, the court ordered the cesarean section. The fetus was indeed to young and too damaged to survive the surgery, and Angela Carder died two days later.

The American Civil Liberties Union (ACLU) took on the case on behalf of the estate of Angela Carder and won, vacating the order and forcing the hospital to pay damages and to acknowledge its error in forcing her to undergo surgery against her will.

While among the most famous, this is assuredly not the only case in which hospitals have declared a right to intervene and do unwanted procedures, including surgery, on pregnant women "in the interest of the fetus." A study in the 1980s found over 20 such cases of forced cesarean sections. The NAPW was founded to protect the rights of pregnant people to make their own medical and health care decisions and not to be treated simply as housing for a fetal patient. Lynn Paltrow filed the first civil rights challenge to a hospital policy of searching pregnant people for drug-use evidence and then turning that information over to the police. That case went to the Supreme Court, where Paltrow successfully argued that such a policy violates the rights of individuals against unreasonable searches and seizures—claiming, in essence, that a pregnant person is a person, with full bodily autonomy and the full rights a person has before the law.

There are five primary concerns the NAPW addresses. The first is that no one is punished for the outcome of their pregnancies. This is the case whether they have an abortion, experience a pregnancy loss, or go to term and give birth to a baby. Second, they are committed to seeing that no one loses their constitutional and human rights by becoming pregnant. Third, they want health and welfare problems people confront in pregnancy, such as addiction, to be attended to as health/medical issues and not as crimes. Fourth, they work to prevent families from being needlessly separated. Fifth, and finally, they want to make sure that pregnant and parenting people have access to a full range of reproductive health care as well as access to confidential, nonpunitive drug treatment services. The NAPW works to achieve this by providing pro bono (no expense) legal services as needed as well as working to educate the public and legislatures.

National Association of Certified Professional Midwives

The National Association of Certified Professional Midwives (NACPM) is the largest professional membership organization for certified professional midwives (CPMs). Founded in 2000, NACPM ensures a powerful and collective voice for CPMs. To date, there are approximately 3,839 CPMs. The NACPM directs its influence toward improving outcomes for childbearing people and their infants, developing and strengthening the profession, and informing public policy with the values inherent in CPM care.

Some of NACPM's commitments include safeguarding the right to normal physiologic birth for every childbearing person; establishing licensure and equitable reimbursement for CPMs in all 50 states, territories, and the District of Columbia; advocating for CPMs to the public, state, and federal legislators and health policy makers; investing in a strong racially, ethnically, and socially representative CPM workforce to meet the needs of childbearing people; eliminating unconscionable disparities in birth outcomes for people of color, Indigenous people, and their infants; dismantling systemic racism in midwifery and the birth care system; opposing the oppression of childbearing women, including the impacts of sexism, misogyny, and gender-based and obstetrical violence; opposing the oppression of LGBTQIA2S+ childbearing people, including homophobia, transphobia, biphobia, and violence based on sexuality, gender expression, and family structure; utilizing NACPM's colonial privilege as an organization to influence policy that recognizes the inherent sovereignty and self-determination of Indigenous peoples; and understanding and addressing the compound negative impact of oppression on childbearing people with multiple intersecting identities. NACPM is a member of the United States Midwifery Education, Regulation, and Association (US MERA) and the International Confederation of Midwives (ICM).

National Association to Advance Black Birth

The National Association to Advance Black Birth (NAABB) began in 1991. It was first founded by Shafia Monroe (see entry in this chapter) as the International Center for Traditional Childbearing (ICTC). The nonprofit organization that Monroe established was dedicated to both building community among birth workers of color, especially Black birth workers, and training doulas. Her vision led to a community of birth workers of color across the country. The language of "traditional childbearing" referred to the history of Black and Indigenous midwives as providing the care of birthing people and families in their communities. The organization states that the vision in its founding was that "there be a midwife for every community, a healthy baby born to every family and the midwife as the norm for women of color." Monroe retired from the organization in 2016.

And after a period of reflection, the new board moved its focus serving the needs of the Black birthing community through advocacy, policy, and scholarship. Accordingly, in 2018, the ICTC changed its name. It also moved its headquarters from Monroe's home base in Portland, Oregon, to Washington, DC.

In its ongoing advocacy work, NAABB works to lend "voice, agency and liberation to Black mothers, children and families," acknowledging that these are people whose experiences are often unseen and unheard due to the legacy, remnants, and ongoing realities of institutionalized racism in American medicine and health systems.

The organization works to achieve its goals through a variety of platforms, including documentary films, speaker presentations and consultations, scholarships to aid African-descent midwifery students, and by making available a Black Birthing Bill of Rights (https://thenaabb.org/index.php/black-birthing-bill-of-rights/).

NAABB is a member of the United States Midwifery Education, Regulation, and Association (US MERA).

National Birth Equity Collaborative

The National Birth Equity Collaborative creates solutions that optimize Black maternal and infant health through training, policy advocacy, research, and community-centered collaboration. NBEC was founded by Dr. Joia Crear-Perry, an obstetrician and policy expert on racism as a root cause of health inequities. NBEC supports collaborative perinatal and reproductive health research through its Birth Equity Research Scholars Program; drafts important policy watch briefs with up-to-date information on legislation and policy impacting perinatal and reproductive health; and, provides training and technical assistance to organizations, communities, and stakeholders. In 2020, NBEC released *The Birth Equity Agenda: A Blueprint for Reproductive Health and Wellbeing*.

National Black Midwives Alliance

The National Black Midwives Alliance (NBMA) was launched by midwives Haguerenesh Tesfa and Jamarah Amani on March 8, 2018, the International Day of the Woman. It is the only professional association of Black midwives in the United States. Its goal is to honor, celebrate, and uplift Black midwives and to have a representative voice that clearly outlines the various needs of Black midwives. The alliance was founded on three pillars that guide its mission: legacy, power, and voice. The NBMA honors the history and traditions of Black midwives and recognizes their power as central community figures and leaders.

Some of the NBMA's objectives are to increase the number of Black midwives and access to Black midwifery care to improve perinatal health disparities; raise public awareness about Black midwives, past and present; support legislative efforts led by Black midwives; advocate for and support the development of educational pathways and mentorship for Black student midwives; and offer continuing education to practicing Black midwives.

The NBMA regularly collaborates with other birth justice and midwifery groups working toward equity and justice within and across maternity care.

Courtesy of Haguerenesh Tesfa

Our Bodies Ourselves

The organization that came to be known as Our Bodies Ourselves began at a 1969 workshop that brought together 12 women from the Boston area who were part of a seminar organized by Nancy Miriam Hawley at Emmanuel College. This was very early in what became known as second-wave feminism and the start of consciousness-raising groups. Women gathered together to learn from each other and to talk about their experiences with their own bodies, health, and sexuality.

In those days, before the internet, information about the body was understood as a very esoteric form of knowledge that only physicians could truly understand and teach. These women, in a spirit most young people of today would recognize, wanted to go past medical expertise and learn from each other. Rather than the very male, patriarchal perspective that medicine brought, these women centered their questions on what women feel, experience, and do.

They came together to write a book, which they printed off on copy machines and sold for 35 cents. That book, *Our Bodies, Ourselves,* had chapters on women's sexuality, contraception, abortion, and what were then called "venereal diseases" as well as the concluding chapters "Medical Institutions" and "Women, Medicine and Capitalism." Chapters on pregnancy are very medically focused, and the chapter on childbirth, called "Prepared Childbirth," discusses the Lamaze technique for managing hospital births.

The women were young and so was the women's movement and what became known as the women's health movement. On the table of contents page of the second edition (1971), they state, "The first printing sold so fast we haven't had time to revise the printed course. . . . We want to add chapters on menopause and getting older and attitudes to children (child rearing alternatives, single women having children, adopting, also not having children). We want to expand the existing chapters to include more on monogamy, homosexuality, women's disease and hysterectomies, the relation between mental and physical health, nutrition, etc." They then asked readers to write up their own experiences and to step up and join them in working on the course.

This 136-page booklet moved on to be published first by Simon and Schuster as a 276-page book in 1973 and eventually to be translated and adapted into 29 languages, selling over four million copies by its final edition in 2011. More specific books were also published, including one focused on pregnancy and childbirth.

Planned Parenthood

Planned Parenthood began as the first clinic in the United States to offer birth control education. It was founded as the American Birth Control League by Margaret Sanger in 1921, five years after opening her Brooklyn Clinic (see Margaret Sanger entry).

In 1942, the organization changed to its current name, Planned Parenthood. This emphasis on parenthood as a planned, chosen state very much represents the modern American cultural perspective. The name shows that the point is not to avoid having babies but to plan one's babies. The emphasis switches from *contraception*, which means "against conception," to a more thoughtful and planned conception. By that point, there were hundreds of Planned Parenthood clinics throughout the United States. Planned Parenthood Federation largely relied on volunteer labor to do what is now called "family planning" counseling.

By the 1970s, with the sexual revolution, second-wave feminism, and the invention of the birth control pill, contraception became a more widely accepted and openly discussed part of American life. It also became more medicalized, with physicians controlling access to more and more contraception. While condoms can still be purchased directly, most of the birth control available for the use of women—then and now—required a medical prescription, including the diaphragm, the various hormonal pills, and the intrauterine device (IUD). Alan Guttmacher, an ob-gyn, served as president of Planned Parenthood from 1962 until his death in 1964. He worked with the International Planned Parenthood Federation as the chair of its Medical Committee and traveled around the world to Asian, African, and Latin American nations to lecture physicians and work with national leaders to make contraception more widely available.

Birth control remained the primary mission, but Planned Parenthood also became a national voice in the abortion discussion, advocating for access to safe abortion care. As contraception became normalized and most physicians became quite comfortable prescribing contraception even for younger people, Planned Parenthood became better known for its provision of abortion services. In the United States, about half of all Planned Parenthood clinics offer abortion services, but all offer contraception and related services, including screening and treatment for sexually transmitted diseases, pregnancy testing, prenatal care, vasectomies and treatment for erectile dysfunction.

Planned Parenthood clinics see approximately three million patients a year in the United States.

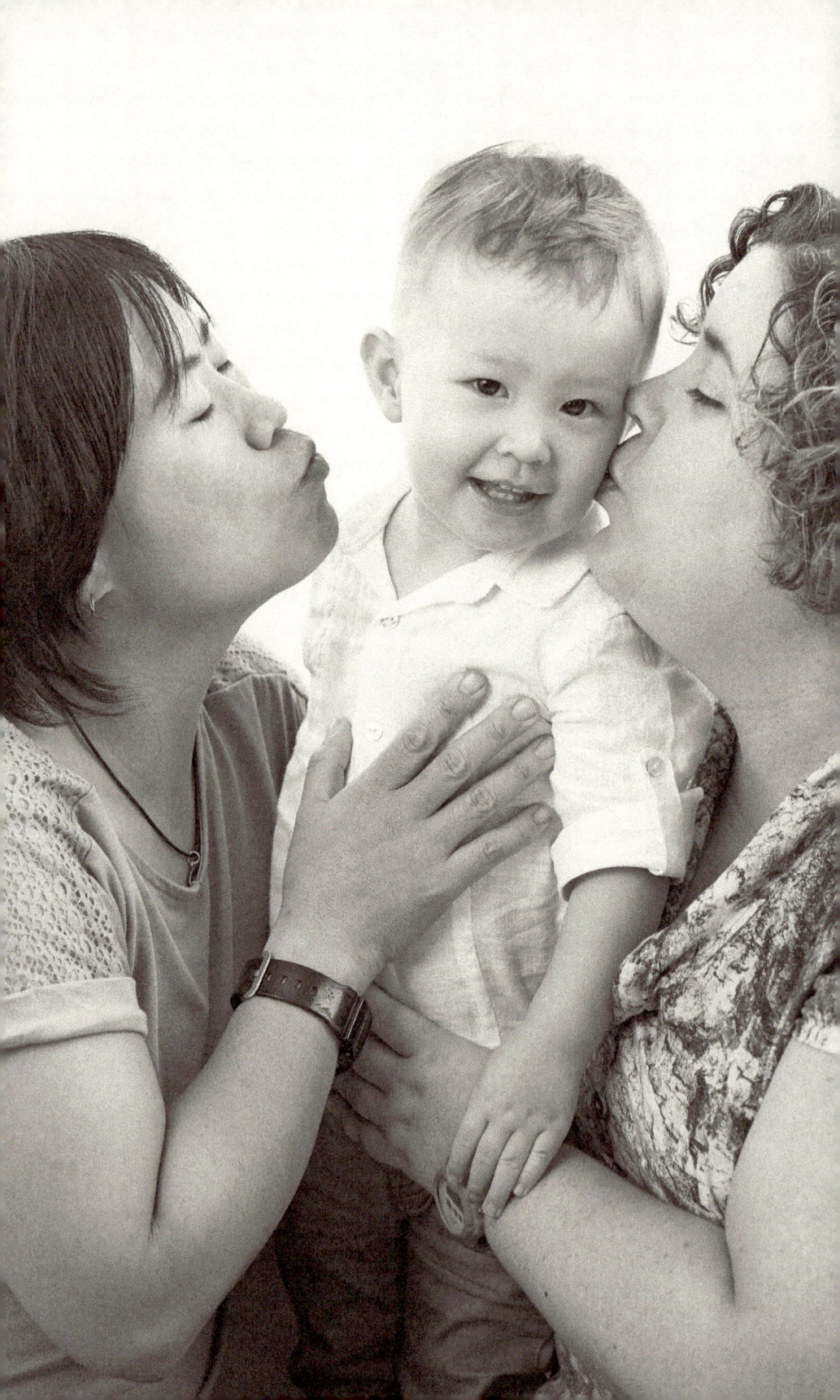

The data in this chapter illustrate the variability in provider state restrictions, the shifts over time in pregnancy and birth outcomes and experiences, and the racial and ethnic disparities among pregnant and birthing people in the United States. The artifacts pertaining to pregnancy and birth in the United States found in this chapter include select historical documents presented in chronological order. These primary texts, created by professional associations, activists, lawmakers, government agencies, and scholars, help situate the conversation within a broader historical context.

Live Births Data

Births and Fertility Rate

The number of births in the United States has consistently fallen between the years of 2007 and 2017 (with the exception of 2014, when birth rates rose). In 2017, there were 3,855,500 births in the United States. The general fertility rate in the United States was 60.3 births per 1,000 people. This is the record low general fertility rate in the United States and down 2 percent from 2016.

The birth rate for people between the ages of 10 and 14 remained unchanged from 2016. The number of births to people between the ages of 15 and 39 decreased 7 percent between 2016 and 2017. For people in their twenties across all racial

---

Parents kissing their child's cheeks. (Dragonimages/Dreamstime.com)

groups, there was a decrease in births. People in their late twenties experienced a lower birth rate than people in their early thirties for the second time since reliable data has been recorded, according to the Centers for Disease Control and Prevention (CDC). The number of births for people between the ages of 35 and 39 rose 1 percent in 2017. The only groups where the birth rates rose were birthing people over forty, up 2 percent from 2016. In 2017, there were 840 births for people aged 50–64.

First Birth Rate

According to the CDC, in 2017, the first birth rate in the United States was 22.9 births per 1,000 births for birthing people between the ages of 15 and 44. This was a decrease in first births for birthing people in their teens, twenties, and thirties. The only increase for first births rates for birthing people was the group in their late forties, between the ages of 45 and 49.

Infant Mortality Rate

Infant mortality rate—death within the first year of life—is a key indicator of a country's health. Though the infant mortality rate in the United States has been declining, it is still considerably higher than other industrialized countries. In 2017, the infant mortality rate in the United States was 5.8 deaths per 1,000 live births. When disaggregated by race and ethnicity, the rates are staggering, with non-Hispanic Black infants, for example, dying at a rate of 11.4 per 1,000 live births, as compared to 4.9 deaths per 1,000 live births for non-Hispanic white infants. American Indian/Alaska Native, Native Hawaiian/Pacific Islander, and Hispanic infants all experience infant death rates higher than non-Hispanic white infants, with Asian infants being the only cohort to experience a lower comparative rate at 3.6 deaths per 1,000 live births.

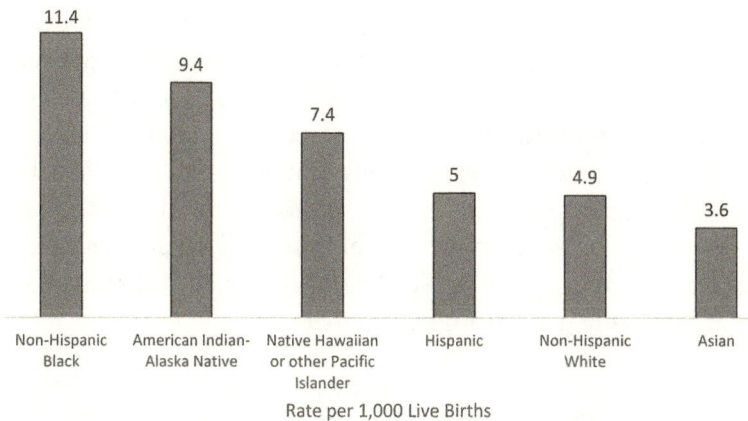

Figure 5.1 Infant Mortality Rate by Race and Ethnicity, 2016

When comparing the United States to other developed countries, the infant mortality rate is higher. For example, as the CDC reports, "after excluding births at less than 24 weeks of gestation to ensure international comparability, the U.S. infant mortality rate was 4.2, still higher than for most European countries and about twice the rates for Finland, Sweden, and Denmark. U.S. infant mortality rates for very preterm infants (24–31 weeks of gestation) compared favorably with most European rates. However, the U.S. mortality rate for infants at 32–36 weeks was second-highest, and the rate for infants at 37 weeks of gestation or more was highest, among the countries studied."

The causes of infant mortality are varied, though intrapartum and postpartum provider care, along with social and structural determinants of health, are essential variables.

Sources: Centers for Disease Control and Prevention. 2020. "Infant Mortality." https://www.cdc.gov/reproductivehealth/maternalinfanthealth/infantmortality.htm#chart; https://www.cdc.gov/nchs/data/nvsr/nvsr63/nvsr63_05.pdf.

Healthy People, an initiative of the Office of Disease Prevention and Health Promotion, provides science-based, 10-year national objectives for improving the health of all Americans. One of the Healthy People 2020 objectives is to reduce infant mortality, or the number of infant deaths per 1,000 live births. This figure illustrates that, in 2018, infant mortality rates were highest among states in the South, though Ohio and West Virginia also have high rates. New Hampshire had the lowest (3.6) and Louisiana had the highest (7.6).

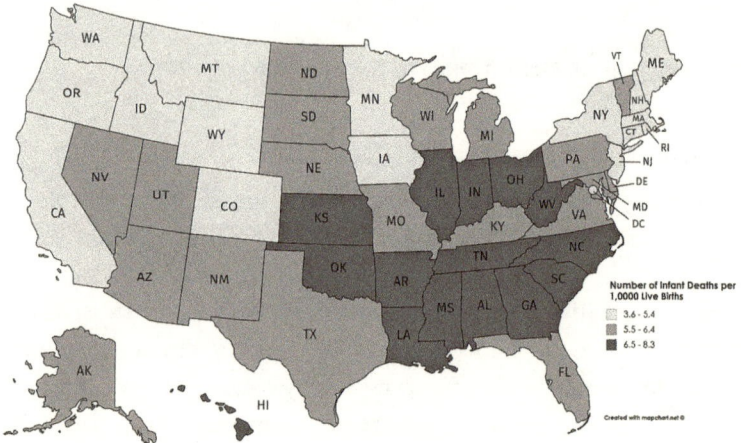

Figure 5.2   Infant Mortality Rate by State, 2018

Source: National Center for Health Statistics. 2020. "Infant Mortality Rates by State." https://www.cdc.gov/nchs/pressroom /sosmap/infant_mortality_rates/infant_mortality.htm.

Maternal Mortality Rate by Race/Ethnicity

One of the most striking indications of perinatal health is the maternal mortality rate (MMR). Pregnant people in the United States are suffering death and injury at increasing rates. According to the CDC, the number of reported pregnancy-related deaths in the United States steadily increased from 7.2 deaths per 100,000 live births in 1987 to 16.9 deaths per 100,000 live births in 2016.

The United States is the only country with an advanced economy where the MMR is getting worse, and it is one of only 13 countries worldwide with a rising MMR. Though the overall proportion of people who do not survive pregnancy and child-bearing is on the rise, birthing people of color are at a much higher risk of maternity-related death and illness. In particular, Black people are dying at a rate three to four times higher than white people. In some American cities, the MMR rate for Black people is higher than in many developing countries.

According to the CDC's Pregnancy Mortality Surveillance System (PMSS), considerable racial/ethnic disparities in pregnancy-related mortality exist. During 2011–2016, the pregnancy-related mortality ratios were 42.4 deaths per 100,000 live births for Black non-Hispanic people; 30.4 deaths per 100,000 live births for American Indian/Alaskan Native non-Hispanic people; 14.1 deaths per 100,000 live births for Asian/Pacific Islander non-Hispanic people; 13.0 deaths per 100,000 live births for white non-Hispanic people; and 11.3 deaths per 100,000 live births for Hispanic people.

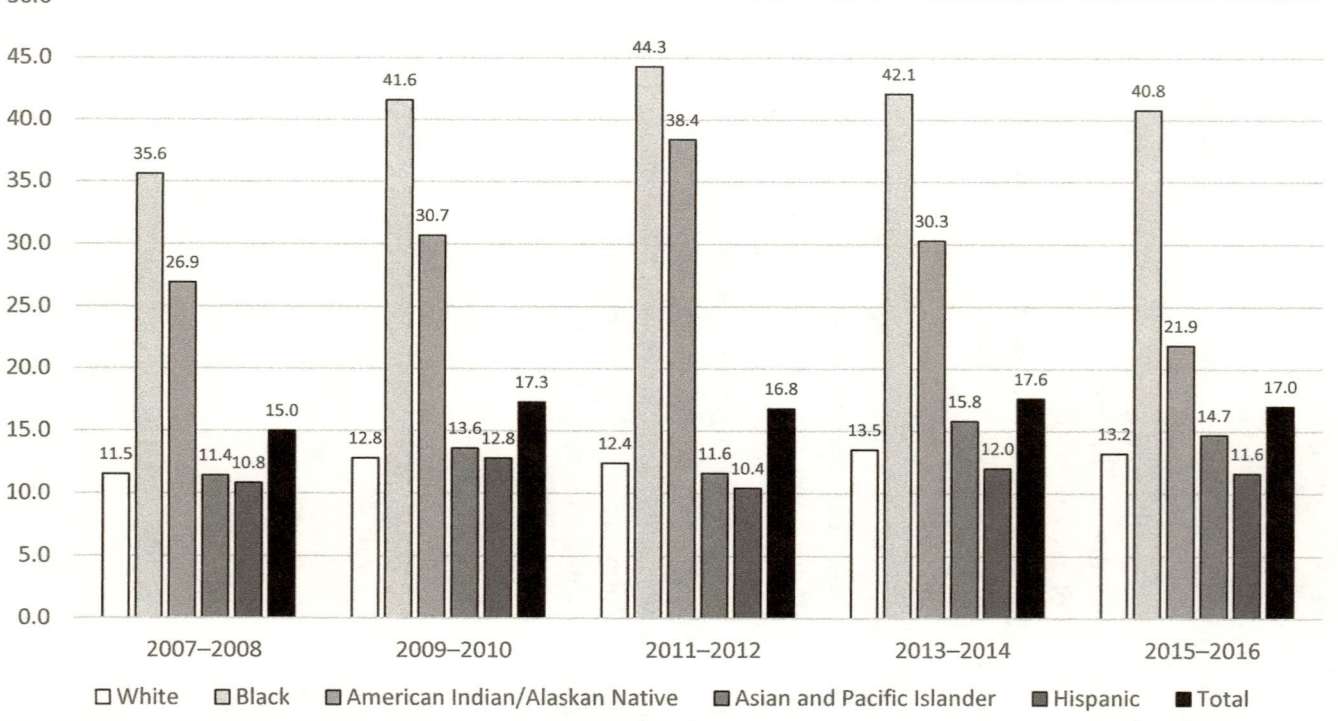

Figure 5.3 Maternal Mortality Rate by Race/Ethnicity, 2007–2016

Source: Petersen, E. E., N. L. Davis, D. Goodman, S. Cox, C. Syverson, K. Seed, C. Shapiro-Mendoza, W. M. Callaghan, and W. Barfield. 2019. "Racial/Ethnic Disparities in Pregnancy-Related Deaths—United States, 2007–2016." *Morbidity and Mortality Weekly Report* 68(35): 762–765. http://dx.doi.org/10.15585/mmwr.mm6835a3.

Birth Rate by State/Region

According to the CDC, during 2007–2017, total fertility rates in the United States fell for rural and metropolitan counties: 12 percent and 16–18 percent, respectively. Rural areas have persistently higher fertility and worse birth outcomes compared with metropolitan areas. Declines in total fertility rates and increases in mean maternal age were also observed for people of each race and Hispanic-origin group, non-Hispanic white, non-Hispanic Black, and Hispanic, by urbanization level from 2007 to 2017. The mean age at first birth was lower for each race and Hispanic-origin group in rural counties than in metropolitan counties.

The general fertility rate declined from 2016 to 2017 by 1–3 percent in 27 states and by 4–6 percent in 14 states and Washington, DC (Alaska, Arizona, California, Colorado, Kansas, Montana, New Mexico, North Dakota, Oklahoma, Oregon, Texas, Utah, Washington, and Wyoming) and was essentially unchanged in 9 states (Alabama, Delaware, Mississippi, New Hampshire, Rhode Island, South Dakota, Tennessee, Vermont, and West Virginia). Rates among the states ranged from 49.7 births per 1,000 females aged 15–44 in Vermont to 76.4 in South Dakota. In 2017, the birth rate for teenagers aged 15–19 declined in 32 states and DC, with declines ranging from 5 percent to 20 percent, and rates were essentially unchanged in the remaining 18 states (Connecticut, Delaware, Hawaii, Idaho, Indiana, Kansas, Maine, Massachusetts, Minnesota, Missouri, Nebraska, New Hampshire, Rhode Island, South Dakota, Utah, Vermont, Virginia, and Wyoming). Rates among the states ranged from 8.1 births per 1,000 in Massachusetts to 32.8 in Arkansas.

Source: Martin, J. A., B. E. Hamilton, M. J. K. Osterman, and A. K. Driscoll. 2018. "Births: Final Data for 2017." National Vital Statistics Reports. https://www.cdc.gov/nchs/data/nvsr /nvsr67/nvsr67_08-508.pdf.

Cesarean Rate

The general cesarean delivery rate, primary cesarean delivery rate, and the low-risk cesarean delivery rate all increased from 2016 to 2017 according to data from the CDC. The general cesarean delivery rate increased to 32.0 percent in 2017 from 31.9 percent in 2016. The primary cesarean delivery rate (cesarean deliveries among people who have not had a previous cesarean delivery) was 21.9 percent, up from 21.8 percent in 2016. The low-risk cesarean delivery rate also increased to 26.0 percent in 2017 from 25.7 percent for 2016. VBAC, or vaginal births after cesarean delivery, rose slightly to 12.8 percent, up 0.4 percent from 12.4 in 2016.

Among the three largest race and Hispanic-origin groups, the cesarean delivery rate increased for Hispanic people from 2016 to 2017 (31.7 percent to 31.8 percent); rates for non-Hispanic white (30.9 percent) and non-Hispanic Black (36.0 percent) people were essentially unchanged.

Source: Martin, J. A., B. E. Hamilton, M. J. K. Osterman, and A. K. Driscoll. 2018. "Births: Final Data for 2017." National Vital Statistics Reports. https://www.cdc.gov/nchs/data/nvsr /nvsr67/nvsr67_08-508.pdf.

Source of Payment

In 2017, most births in the United States were covered by private insurance or Medicaid. Private insurance payments declined from 49.4 percent in 2016 to 49.1 percent in 2017. Medicare birth payments rose from 42.6 percent in 2016 to 43 percent in 2017.

Medicaid coverage for birth increased for each of the three largest race and Hispanic-origin groups during 2016–2017. In

2017, Medicaid-covered births ranged from 30.5 percent for non-Hispanic white people to 65.9 percent for non-Hispanic Black people. The percentage of birth payments by private insurance declined from 2016 to 2017 for non-Hispanic white people, from 63.3 percent to 63.1 percent. Private insurance payments increased for Hispanic people, from 28.4 percent to 28.5 percent, and remained unchanged for non-Hispanic Black people at 27.7 percent in 2017.

Source: Martin, J. A., B. E. Hamilton, M. J. K. Osterman, and A. K. Driscoll. 2018. "Births: Final Data for 2017." National Vital Statistics Reports. https://www.cdc.gov/nchs/data/nvsr/nvsr67/nvsr67_08-508.pdf.

Period of Gestation

The preterm birth rate (percentage of all births delivered at less than 37 completed weeks of gestation) in the United States rate rose to 9.93 percent in 2017, nearly a 1 percent rise from 9.85 percent in 2016. This was the third straight year of increases in the U.S. preterm birth rate since 2014, when it was 9.57 percent. The preterm birth rate had been declining steadily from 10.44 percent in 2007. Most of the increase in the total preterm birth rate for 2016–2017 was among infants born late preterm (34–36 weeks), up from 7.09 percent to 7.17 percent. The early preterm birth rate (less than 34 weeks) was 2.76 percent in 2017, which was unchanged since 2015 but down from 2.93 percent in 2007. The percentage of infants born early term (37–38 weeks) rose by 2 percent in 2017, from 25.47 percent to 26.00 percent. The full-term (39–40 weeks) birth rate declined from 57.94 percent to 57.49 percent in 2017.

In contrast, from 2007 to 2014, the early term birth rate had generally been on the decline, and the full-term rate had been on the rise. Declines were also seen from 2016 to 2017 in late (41 weeks) and post-term (42 and higher) births. Preterm birth rates among non-Hispanic white birthing people were essentially unchanged between 2016 and 2017 at 9.05 percent.

Preterm birth rates rose among non-Hispanic Black, from 13.77 percent to 13.93 percent, and Hispanic (9.45 percent to 9.62 percent) birthing people. For 2017, preterm birth rates for the three major race and Hispanic-origin groups ranged from a high of 13.93 percent among non-Hispanic Black birthing people to a low of 8.53 percent among non-Hispanic Asian birthing people. Preterm levels for the Hispanic subgroups varied, ranging from 9.05 percent for Cubans to 11.20 percent for Puerto Ricans.

Source: Martin, J. A., B. E. Hamilton, M. J. K. Osterman, and A. K. Driscoll. 2018. "Births: Final Data for 2017." National Vital Statistics Reports. https://www.cdc.gov/nchs/data/nvsr/nvsr67/nvsr67_08-508.pdf.

Birthweight

In 2017, the percentage of infants born low birth weight (LBW) rose for the third year in a row to 8.28 percent from 8.17 percent in 2016. The LBW rate (the percentage of infants born weighing less than 2,500 grams or 5 pounds, 8 ounces) has risen 4 percent since the most recent low in 2014 (8 percent) and is the highest rate reported since the 2006 peak (8.26 percent). From 1990 to 2006, LBW levels rose nearly 20 percent but then declined from 2007 to 2012 (7.99 percent). The percentage of infants born with very low birthweight (VLBW, less than 1,500 grams) was essentially unchanged at 1.41 percent in 2017 compared with 1.40 percent in 2016. The VLBW rate has essentially been stable at 1.40–1.41 percent since 2013, but it is down from a high of 1.49 percent for 2005–2007. The percentage of moderately low birthweight infants (1,500–2,499 grams) increased from 6.77 percent in 2016 to 6.87 percent in 2017, surpassing the peak reported for 2006 (6.77 percent). Between 2016 and 2017, LBW rates were essentially stable among non-Hispanic white people (6.97 percent to 7.00 percent), but rates rose slightly for births to non-Hispanic Black

(13.68 percent to 13.89 percent) and Hispanic (7.32 percent to 7.43 percent) people.

The LBW rate among singleton births only rose from 6.44 percent to 6.56 percent from 2016 to 2017. As with LBW among all births, the increase was predominantly for infants born with a moderately low birth weight. It can be informative to examine births in singleton deliveries separately because multiple births tend to be born smaller than singletons, and changes in multiple-birth incidence can influence overall LBW levels.

Source: Martin, J. A., B. E. Hamilton, M. J. K. Osterman, and A. K. Driscoll. 2018. "Births: Final Data for 2017." National Vital Statistics Reports. https://www.cdc.gov/nchs/data/nvsr /nvsr67/nvsr67_08-508.pdf.

Multiple Births

The 2017 twin birth rate was 33.3 twins per 1,000 births. The twinning rate (births in twin deliveries per 1,000 total births) rose 76 percent from 1980 to 2009 (from 18.9 to 33.2 per 1,000). It was generally stable from 2009 through 2012 and then rose for 2013 and 2014; the 2014 rate of 33.9 was the highest ever reported. The triplet and higher-order multiple birth rate (triplet/+) was 101.6 per 100,000 births for 2017, which was not statistically different from 2016 (101.4 births per 100,000); the 2016 and 2017 rates are the lowest reported in more than two decades. The triplet/+ birth rate (number of triplets, quadruplets, and quintuplets and other higher-order multiples per 100,000 births) rose more than 400 percent from 1980 to 1998, but it has fallen 47 percent since the 1998 peak of 193.5 per 100,000 birth.

There were 128,310 infants born in twin deliveries in 2017. The number of triplet/+ births in 2017, 3,917, was the lowest number reported in 25 years (since 1992) and about one-half of the highest number reported (7,663 triplet/+ births in 2003). In 2017, triplet/+ births included 3,675 triplet, 193 quadruplet, and 49 quintuplet and higher-order multiple births. Twin birth rates increased among non-Hispanic Black people (from 39.9 to 41.0 per 1,000), but the rates were largely stable among non-Hispanic white (35.7 to 35.5) and Hispanic (24.6 to 24.5) people. Triplet/+ birth rates rose among both non-Hispanic Black (112.4 to 119.7 per 100,000) and Hispanic (58.6 to 68.3) women but declined for non-Hispanic white people (121.7 to 116.6).

Since the first U.S. infant conceived with assisted reproductive technology (ART) was born in 1981, both the use of ART and the number of fertility clinics providing ART services have steadily increased in the United States. ART includes fertility treatments in which eggs or embryos are handled in the laboratory (i.e., in vitro fertilization [IVF] and related procedures). Although the majority of infants conceived through ART are singletons, people who undergo ART procedures are more likely than people who conceive naturally to deliver multiple-birth infants.

Of ART-conceived infants, 35.3 percent were born in multiple-birth deliveries compared with 3.4 percent of all infants. ART-conceived twins accounted for approximately 96.1 percent (22,491 of 23,413) of all ART-conceived infants born in multiple deliveries. ART-conceived multiple-birth infants contributed to 17 percent of all multiple-birth infants. Approximately 33.9 percent of all ART-conceived infants were twins, compared with 3.3 percent of all infants. ART-conceived twins contributed to 16.8 percent of all twins. Finally, 1.4 percent of ART-conceived infants were triplets and higher-order multiples compared with 0.1–0.2 percent of all infants. ART-conceived triplets and higher-order infants contributed to 22.2 percent of all triplets and higher-order infants.

Sources: Centers for Disease Control and Prevention. 2019. "National ART Surveillance." https://www.cdc.gov/art/nass /index.html; Martin, J. A., B. E. Hamilton, M. J. K. Osterman, and A. K. Driscoll. 2018. "Births: Final Data for 2017."

National Vital Statistics Reports. https://www.cdc.gov/nchs /data/nvsr/nvsr67/nvsr67_08-508.pdf.

Abortion/Termination

Abortion care is health care, and an important Reproductive Justice issue. A total of 638,169 abortions for 2015 were reported to CDC from 49 reporting areas. The abortion rate for 2015 was 11.8 abortions per 1,000 women aged 15–44 years, and the abortion ratio was 188 abortions per 1,000 live births. From 2014 to 2015, the total number of reported abortions decreased 2 percent, the abortion rate decreased 2 percent, and the abortion ratio decreased 2 percent. From 2006 to 2015, the total number of reported abortions decreased 24 percent, the abortion rate decreased 26 percent, and the abortion ratio decreased 19 percent. In 2015, all three measures reached their lowest level for the entire period of analysis (2006–2015).

In 2015 and throughout the period of analysis, birthing people in their 20s accounted for the majority of abortions and had the highest abortion rates; birthing people over age 30 accounted for a smaller percentage of abortions and had lower abortion rates. From 2006 to 2015, the abortion rate decreased among birthing people in all age groups. From 2006 to 2015, the percentage of abortions accounted for by adolescents aged 15–19 years decreased 41 percent, and their abortion rate decreased 54 percent. This decrease was greater than the decreases for birthing people in any older age group.

In contrast to the percentage distribution of abortions and abortion rates by age, abortion ratios in 2015 and throughout the entire period of analysis were highest among adolescents and lowest among birthing people aged 25–39 years. Abortion ratios decreased from 2006 to 2015 for birthing people in all age groups.

In 2015, 65.4 percent of abortions were performed at less than 8 weeks' gestation, and 91.1 percent were performed at less than 13 weeks' gestation. Only 7.6 percent of abortions were performed between 14 and 20 weeks' gestation, and only 1.3 percent at greater than 21 weeks' gestation.

In 2015, 24.6 percent of all abortions were performed by early nonsurgical medical abortion, 64.3 percent were performed by surgical abortion at less than 13 weeks' gestation, and 8.8 percent were performed by surgical abortion at greater than 13 weeks' gestation; all other methods were uncommon (less than 2.2 percent). Among those that were eligible for early medical abortion on the basis of being less than 8 weeks' gestation, 35.8 percent were completed by this method.

In 2015, people with one or more previous live births accounted for 59.3 percent of abortions, and people with no previous live births accounted for 40.7 percent. People with one or more previous induced abortions accounted for 43.6 percent of abortions, and people with no previous abortion accounted for 56.3 percent.

Source: Jatlaoui, T. C., L. Eckhaus, M. G. Mandel, A. Nguyen, T. Oduyebo, E. Petersen, and M. K. Whiteman. 2019. "Abortion Surveillance—United States, 2016." *Surveillance Summarie.* https://www.cdc.gov/mmwr/volumes/68/ss/ss6811a1.htm.

Pregnancy Loss Data

Stillbirth

In the United States, a miscarriage is usually defined as loss of a baby before the 20th week of pregnancy, and a stillbirth is the loss of a baby after 20 weeks of pregnancy. Stillbirth is further classified as either early, late, or term. An early stillbirth is a fetal death occurring between 20 and 27 completed weeks of pregnancy. A late stillbirth occurs between 28 and 36 completed weeks of pregnancy. A term stillbirth occurs between 37 or more completed weeks of pregnancy. Stillbirth affects about 1 percent of all pregnancies.

Source: Centers for Disease Control and Prevention. 2020. "What Is Stillbirth?" https://www.cdc.gov/ncbddd/stillbirth/facts.html.

Miscarriage

Miscarriage is when a fetus dies in utero before 20 weeks of pregnancy. For people who know they are pregnant, about 10 to 15 in 100 pregnancies (10–15 percent) end in miscarriage. Most miscarriages happen in the first trimester, before the 12th week of pregnancy. Miscarriage in the second trimester (between 13 and 19 weeks) happens in 1 to 5 in 100 pregnancies (1–5 percent).

As many as half of all pregnancies may end in miscarriage. We do not know the exact number because a miscarriage may happen before a person knows they are pregnant. Many who miscarry may go on to have a healthy pregnancy later if they so choose.

Source: March of Dimes. 2020. "Miscarriage." https://www .marchofdimes.org/complications/miscarriage.aspx.

Provider Data

Midwifery Workforce

There are multiple professional midwifery credentials in the United States (see chapter 1). According to the North American Registry of Midwives, approximately 3,839 CPM credentials have been issued as of 2020. The American Midwifery Certification Board reports 13,074 CNM credentials and 117 CM credentials issued as of 2020. Midwifery, as a profession, is in need of a substantive national workforce analysis.

Source: "Certified Nurse-Midwives/Certified Midwives by State." 2020. https://www.amcbmidwife.org/docs/default -source/default-document-library/number-of-cnm-cm-by -state---august-2020.pdf?sfvrsn=74558eec_0.

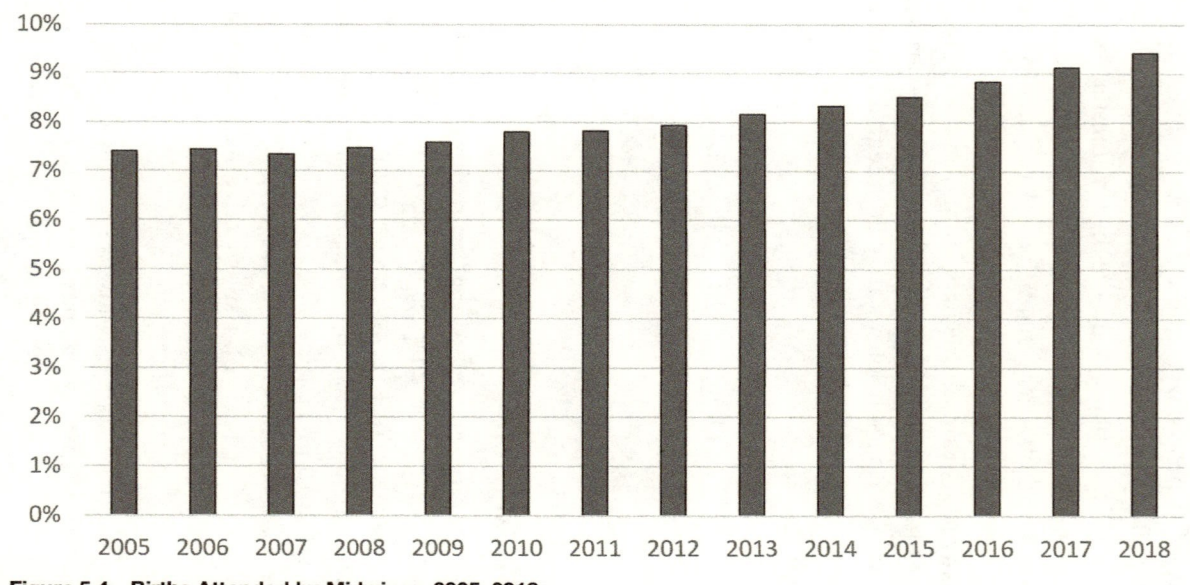

Figure 5.4 Births Attended by Midwives, 2005–2018

Source: Centers for Disease Control and Prevention. "Births: Final Data for 2005 (vol. 56, no. 6), 2006 (vol. 57, no. 7), 2007 (vol. 58, no. 24), 2008 (vol. 59, no. 1), 2009 (vol. 60, no. 1), 2010 (vol. 61, no. 1), 2011 (vol. 62, no. 1), 2012 (vol. 62, no. 9), 2013 (vol. 64, no. 1), 2014 (vol. 64, no. 12), 2015 (vol. 66, no. 1), 2016 (vol. 67, no. 1), 2017 (vol. 67, no. 8), and 2018 (vol. 68, no. 13)." *National Vital Statistics Reports.* https://www.cdc.gov/nchs/products/nvsr.htm.

Table 5.1 Births by Attendant, Place of Delivery, and Race/and Hispanic Origin of Mother: United States, 2018

Place of Delivery and Race and Hispanic Origin of Mother	All Births	Physician				Midwife			Other	Unspecified
		Total	Doctor of Medicine	Doctor of Osteopathy	Total	Certified Nurse-Midwife	Other Midwife			
All Races and Origins[1]										
Total	3,791,712	3,369,567	3,066,477	303,090	387,519	357,297	30,222	32,185	2,441
Not in hospital	62,266	2,615	2,289	326	45,786	21,008	24,778	12,759	1,262
Freestanding birth center	19,871	531	404	127	18,266	11,139	7,127	958	116
Clinic or doctor's office	596	140	125	15	426	305	121	23	7
Residence	38,512	1,416	1,296	120	26,222	9,3399	16,823	10,089	785
Other	3,287	528	464	64	872	165	707	1,689	198
Not specified	247	36	35	1	76	22	54	62	73
In hospital[2]	3,729,199	3,366,916	3,064,153	302,763	341,657	336,267	5,390	19,364	1,262
Non-Hispanic, Single Race[2]										
White:										
Total	1,956,413	1,718,149	1,534,961	183,188	218,770	195,495	23,275	18,265	1,229
Not in hospital	47,957	1,537	1,298	239	37,315	17,163	20,152	8,489	616
Freestanding birth center	15,547	475	357	118	14,203	8,885	5,318	780	89
Clinic or doctor's office	502	88	79	9	400	282	118	10	4
Residence	29,994	712	642	70	21,927	7,881	14,046	6,925	430
Other	1,914	262	220	42	785	115	670	774	93
Not specified	106	18	17	1	50	13	37	22	16
In hospital[2]	1,908,350	1,716,594	1,533,646	182,948	181,405	178,319	3,086	9,754	597

Black:

Total	552,029	501,224	469,168	32,056	45,851	44,163	1,688	4,570	384
Not in hospital	4,190	529	500	29	1,901	944	957	1,606	154
Freestanding birth center	1,110	17	16	1	1,037	595	442	41	15
Clinic or doctor's office	23	17	17	--	4	4	--	2	--
Residence	2,652	364	345	19	840	334	506	1,336	112
Other	405	131	122	9	20	11	9	227	27
Not specified	29	7	7	--	4	1	3	13	5
In hospital[2]	547,810	500,668	468,661	32,027	43,946	43,218	728	2,951	225

Hispanic[3]

Total	886,210	796,921	735,728	61,193	82,999	79,560	3,439	5,815	475
Not in hospital	5,671	317	288	29	3,837	1,587	2,250	1,304	213
Freestanding birth center	2,030	25	23	2	1,923	981	942	76	6
Clinic or doctor's office	31	15	13	2	11	9	2	2	3
Residence	3,142	192	173	19	1,867	578	1,289	932	151
Other	468	85	79	6	36	19	17	294	53
Not specified	51	6	6	--	8	4	4	14	23
In hospital[2]	880,488	796,598	735,434	61,164	79,154	77,969	1,185	4,497	239

[1] Includes births to race and origin groups not shown separately, such as Hispanic single-race white, Hispanic single-race Black, and non-Hispanic multiple-race women, and births with origin not stated.

[2] Includes births occurring en route to or on arrival at hospital

[2] Race and Hispanic origin are reported separately on birth certificates; persons of Hispanic origin may be of any race. In this table, non-Hispanic women are classified by race. Race categories are consistent with the 1997 Office of Management and Budget standards; see Technical Notes in report. Single race is defined as only one race reported on the birth certificate.

[3] Includes all persons of Hispanic origin of any race; see Technical Notes.

Source: Centers for Disease Control and Prevention. 2019. "Births: Final Data for 2018." *National Vital Statistics Reports* 68(13). https://www.cdc.gov/nchs/data/nvsr/nvsr68 _13_tables-508.pdf.

Obstetrics-Gynecology Workforce

The number of American College of Obstetricians and Gynecologists (ACOG) fellows in practice in 2017 was 35,586, including 31,163 fellows and 4,235 junior fellows in active practice. Using U.S. census estimates, the number of ACOG fellows per 10,000 women aged 16 years or older was 2.7 in 2016 (down from 3.1 in 2008) and per 10,000 women of reproductive age (15–44 years) was 5.5 in 2016 (down from 6.2 in 2008). The percentage of women matching into obstetrics-gynecology residency programs continues to increase (82.3 percent in 2016). The percentage of female obstetrician-gynecologists (ob-gyns) is expected to constitute approximately 66 percent of all ob-gyns in the next 10 years. Female physicians are more likely than male physicians to be nonwhite, and ob-gyns are most likely to identify as women. In 2016, ob-gyns were reported to have the highest proportion of people of color (18.4 percent in 2014, combined), especially African Americans (11.1 percent) and Hispanics (6.7 percent). Underrepresented minority ob-gyns are more likely than white or Asian ob-gyns to practice in federally funded underserved areas or in areas where poverty levels are high. American Indians, Alaska Natives, and Pacific Islanders comprise the ob-gyn group with the highest proportion practicing in rural areas. Ob-gyn density is declining in metropolitan and rural areas. Approximately one-half (49 percent) of the 3,143 U.S. counties lacked a single ob-gyn. More than 10 million women (8.2 percent of all women) in the United States lived in designated Health Professional Shortage Areas (HPSAs).

Substantial geographic imbalances exist in the current supply of ob-gyns in the United States. Over the next decade, this demand for services is projected to increase nationally at a modest 6 percent rate. Without increases in the number of obstetric–gynecologic trainees, the nation will rely heavily on services by nonphysician health care professionals. Furthermore, other physicians trained to address many of the general health care needs of people include obstetric–gynecologic subspecialists and family primary care physicians. Forecasted shortfalls in clinical equivalents of physicians suggest that ob-gyns in certain locations may have to limit their practices more and not assume expanded roles in addressing people's primary care needs. Increasing demand for services related to obstetrics and gynecology is anticipated to be highest among underrepresented populations (especially Hispanic people). Figure 5.5 reflects projected shortfalls as of 2020. ACOG projects a shortfall of up to 22,000 ob-gyns by 2050.

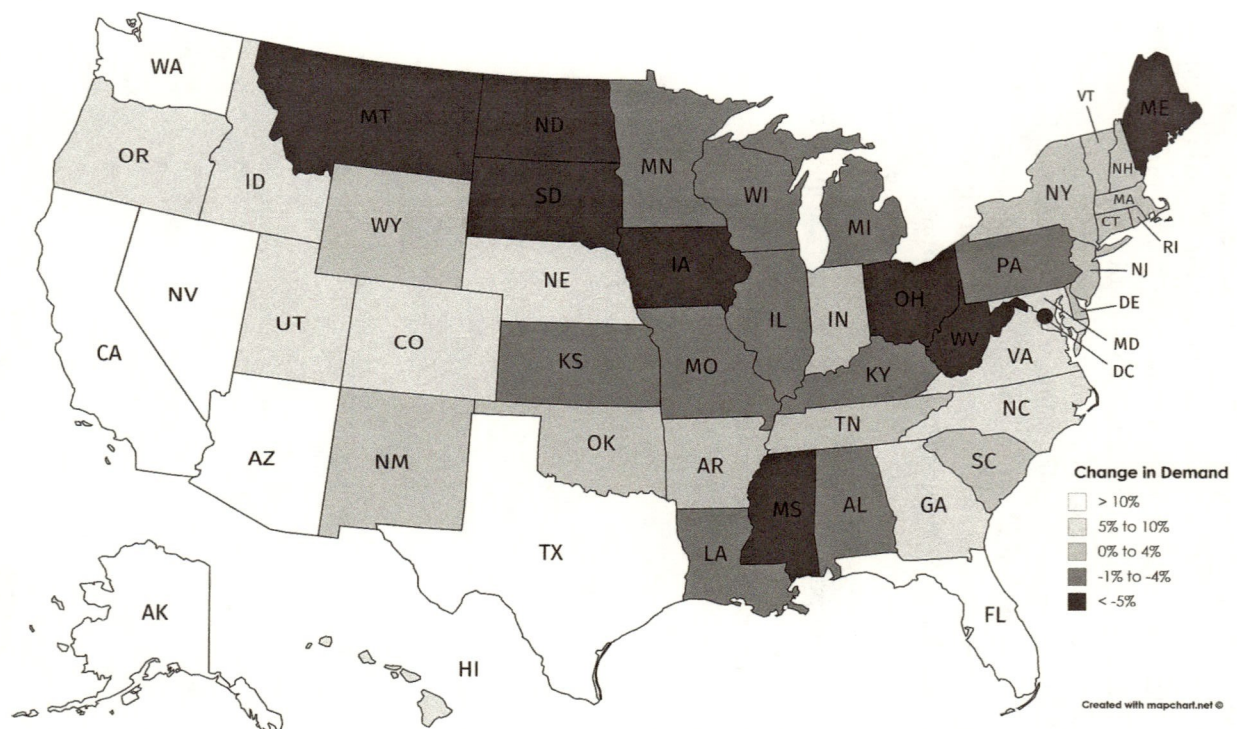

Figure 5.5   Estimated Change in Demand for Perinatal and Women's Health Services, 2020

Change in Demand
> 10%
5% to 10%
0% to 4%
-1% to -4%
< -5%

Sources: https://www.ncbi.nlm.nih.gov/pmc/articles/PMC 3704110/; Rayburn, W. F. 2017. *The Obstetrician-Gynecologists Workforce in the United States: Facts, Figures, and Implications.* 2nd ed. Washington, DC: American College of Obstetricians and Gynecologists; https://s3.amazonaws.com/s3.doximity.com /press/2019_ob_gyn_workforce_study.pdf.

Formative Research

Strong Start for Mothers and Newborns Initiative, 2012–2016

The Strong Start for Mothers and Newborns Initiative was a joint effort between the Centers for Medicare & Medicaid Services (CMS), the Health Resources and Services Administration (HRSA), and the Administration on Children and Families (ACF). The Strong Start for Mothers and Newborns Initiative was a four-year effort by the U.S. Department of Health & Human Services (HHS) that had two strategies to reduce preterm births and improve outcomes for newborns and pregnant people. The first was a public-private partnership and awareness campaign to reduce the rate of early elective deliveries prior to 39 weeks for all populations. The other component was a funding opportunity to test the effectiveness of specific enhanced prenatal care approaches to reduce the frequency of premature births among pregnant Medicaid or Children's Health Insurance Program (CHIP) beneficiaries at high risk for preterm births.

This effort tested ways to encourage best practices and support providers in reducing early elective deliveries prior to 39 weeks. CMS also teamed up with advocacy and professional organizations to increase public awareness efforts and develop new ones. This initiative tested three evidence-based maternity care service approaches that enhanced care delivery and addressed the medical, behavioral, and psychosocial factors that might be present during pregnancy and contribute to preterm-related poor birth outcomes. The 27 awardees tested one of three interventions for enhanced prenatal care, either through centering/group visits, at birth centers, or at maternity care homes.

This initiative builds on decades of work by organizations such as ACOG, the March of Dimes, the National Partnership for Women and Families, the Society for Maternal-Fetal Medicine, and Childbirth Connection, showing that elective deliveries before 39 weeks increase the risk of significant complications for both the birthing person and the baby as well as long-term health problems.

People who received prenatal care in Strong Start birth centers had better birth outcomes and lower costs relative to similar Medicaid beneficiaries not enrolled in Strong Start. In particular, rates of preterm birth, low birth weight, and cesarean section were lower among birth center participants, and costs were more than $2,000 lower per parent-infant pair during birth and the following year.

Table 5.2   Outcomes for Strong Start Participants Relative to Similar Medicaid Participants

	Maternity Care Homes	Group Prenatal Care	Birth Centers
Definition	Enhanced prenatal care including psychosocial support, education, and health promotion in addition to traditional prenatal care. Services provided expanded access to care, improved care coordination, and provided a broader array of health services.	Group prenatal care that incorporated peer-to-peer interaction in a facilitated setting for health assessment, education, and psychosocial support.	Comprehensive prenatal care facilitated by teams of health professionals including peer counselors. Services included collaborative practice, intensive case management, counseling, and psychosocial support.
Costs	Higher costs through delivery period and following year	$427 lower per person during eight months before birth	$2,010 lower through birth and year following for each parent-child pair

(continued)

Table 5.2 *(continued)*

	Maternity Care Homes	Group Prenatal Care	Birth Centers
Utilization	• Fewer prenatal hospitalizations • More infant emergency department visits and hospitalizations	• Fewer emergency department visits and hospitalizations for parent and infant	• Fewer infant emergency department visits and hospitalizations
Quality*	• Higher rate of low birth weight • More weekend deliveries	• Lower very low birth weight rate • More weekend deliveries • More VBACs	• Lower low birth weight rate • Lower preterm birth rate • More weekend deliveries • More VBACs • Fewer C-sections

*Weekend deliveries indicate fewer scheduled inductions and scheduled C-sections. VBAC = vaginal birth after cesarean.

Source: "Strong Start for Mothers and Newborns Initiative: General Information." 2020. https://innovation.cms.gov/initiatives /strong-start.

The Giving Voice to Mothers Study and the Mothers on Respect Index

In the Giving Voice to Mothers Study, community members worked with researchers to design a survey that would capture their lived experiences of care during pregnancy and childbirth, including mistreatment by health providers or health systems. Researchers collected information across the country, including from communities of color and women who planned to give birth at home or in a birthing center. Of the 2,700 women-identifying people who filled out the survey, one in six (17.3 percent) reported mistreatment. Being shouted at or scolded by a health care provider was the most commonly reported type of mistreatment (8.5 percent) followed by "health care providers ignoring women, refusing their request for help, or failing to respond to requests for help in a reasonable amount of time" (7.8 percent). Some women reported violations of physical privacy (5.5 percent) and health care providers threatening to withhold treatment or forcing them to accept treatment they did not want (4.5 percent). Women of color, women who gave birth in hospitals, and those who faced social, economic, or health challenges reported higher rates of mistreatment. Rates were also increased in women who had unexpected events, such as a cesarean or a transfer from community to hospital care, and women who disagreed with a health care provider about the right care for themselves or the baby reported the highest rates of mistreatment.

While significant disparities in maternal and newborn outcomes are reported across populations in the United States, very little is known about whether mistreatment is a component of these adverse outcomes. To understand experiences of childbirth care, especially among communities of color and those who choose to deliver in community settings, service users partnered with nongovernmental organizations (NGOs), clinicians, and researchers to conduct the Giving Voice to Mothers (GVtM) U.S. study.

To date, evaluations of respectful maternity care (RMC) have primarily focused on monitoring care during hospital births in low-resource settings. However, childbearing women from high- and middle-resource countries have also reported negative experiences during hospital births, including being ignored, belittled, or verbally humiliated by health care providers; having interventions forced upon them; and being separated from their babies without reason or explanation. In high-resource countries, pregnant people who are recent immigrants, Indigenous, or disenfranchised by their lower socioeconomic status, race/ethnicity, incarceration, substance dependence, or housing instability have been reported to be at increased risk for poor health outcomes and reduced access to high-quality care.

The GVtM U.S. study led to the development of several new patient-designed indicators of mistreatment in maternity care. The study captured the lived experience from the service user's perspective and could be used to quantify the nature and frequency of occurrence of different types of disrespect and abuse. The indicators are closely aligned with global definitions of the domains of mistreatment and thus are relevant across high-, middle-, and low-resource countries. With some translation and adaptation, these indicators could be implemented in patient-reported outcomes research globally. In the United States, these indicators could be incorporated as performance measures to incentivize expansion of programs to address settings, practices, and institutional cultures that lead to persistent disparities in maternity care.

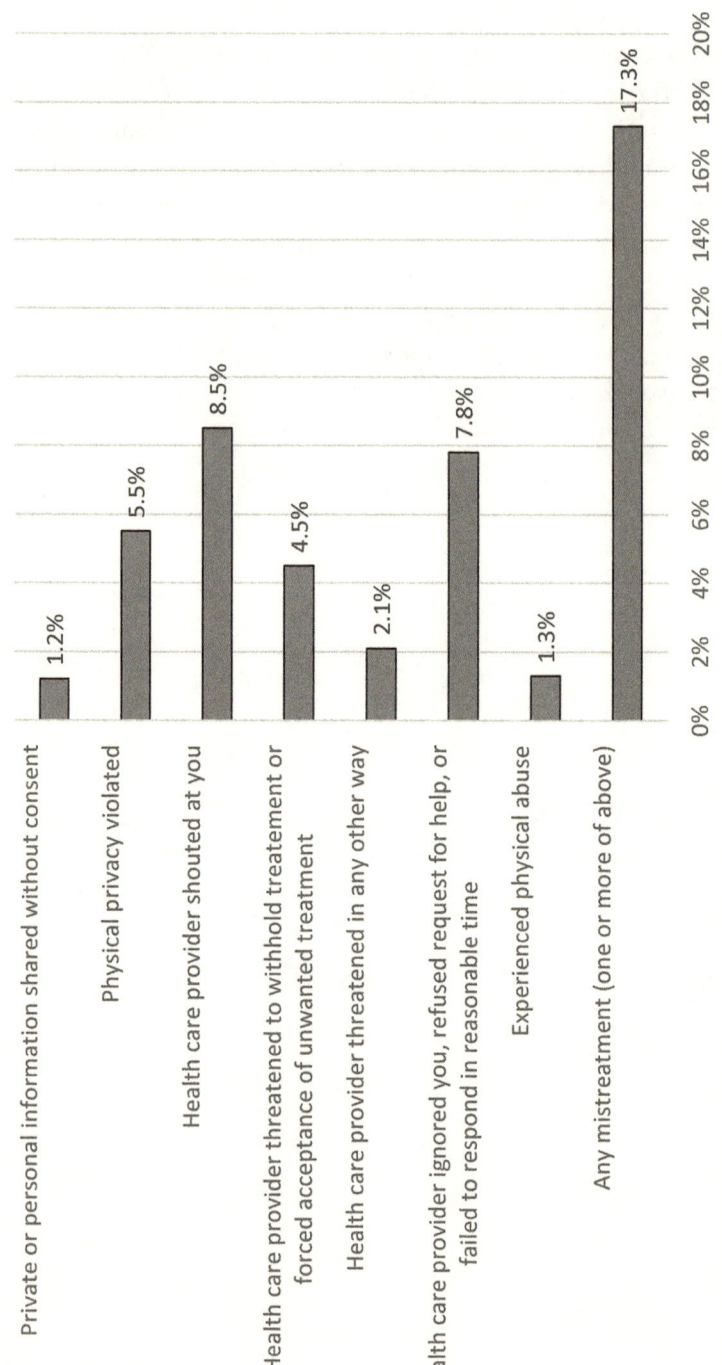

Figure 5.6 Mistreatment by Care Providers in Childbirth

Source: Vedam, S., K. Stoll, N. Rubashkin, K. Martin, Z. Miller-Vedam, H. Hayes-Klein, and G. Jolicoeur. 2017. "The Mothers on Respect (MOR) Index: Measuring Quality, Safety, and Human Rights in Childbirth." *SSM—Population Health* 3: 201–210. https://doi.org/10.1016/j.ssmph.2017.01.005.

Mapping Integration of Midwives across the United States

The Midwifery Integration Scoring System (MISS) assesses the level of integration of midwives and evaluates regional access to high-quality maternity care. In the United States, higher MISS scores were associated with significantly higher rates of physiologic birth, less obstetric interventions, and fewer adverse neonatal outcomes.

Poor coordination of care across providers and birth settings has been associated with adverse maternal-newborn outcomes. Research suggests that the integration of midwives into regional health systems is a key determinant of optimal maternal-newborn outcomes; yet, to date, the characteristics of an integrated system have not been described nor linked to health disparities.

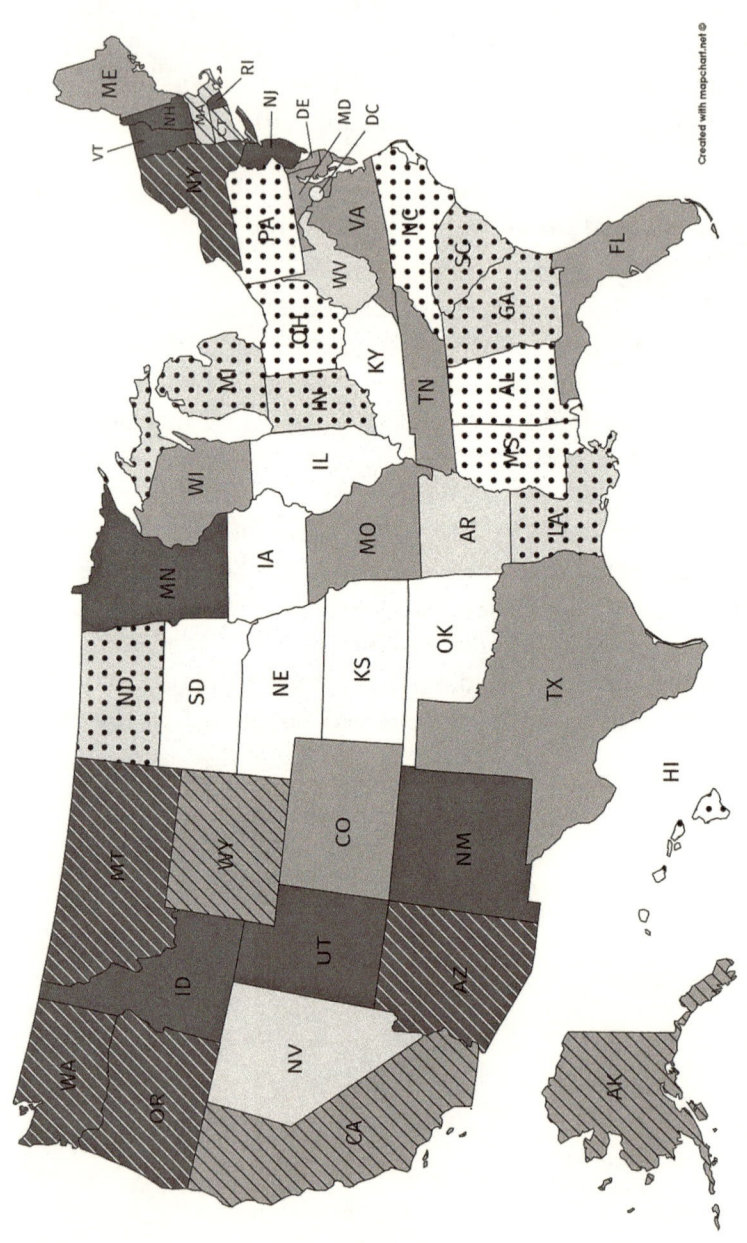

Figure 5.7 Mapping of Integration of Midwives in the United States

Map A: Levels of integration displayed by quartiles of MISS scores. Deeper shades of gray represent higher integration and lighter shades represent lower integration of midwives. States with diagonal lines show where rates of neonatal mortality are lowest, and states with dots show where rates are highest.

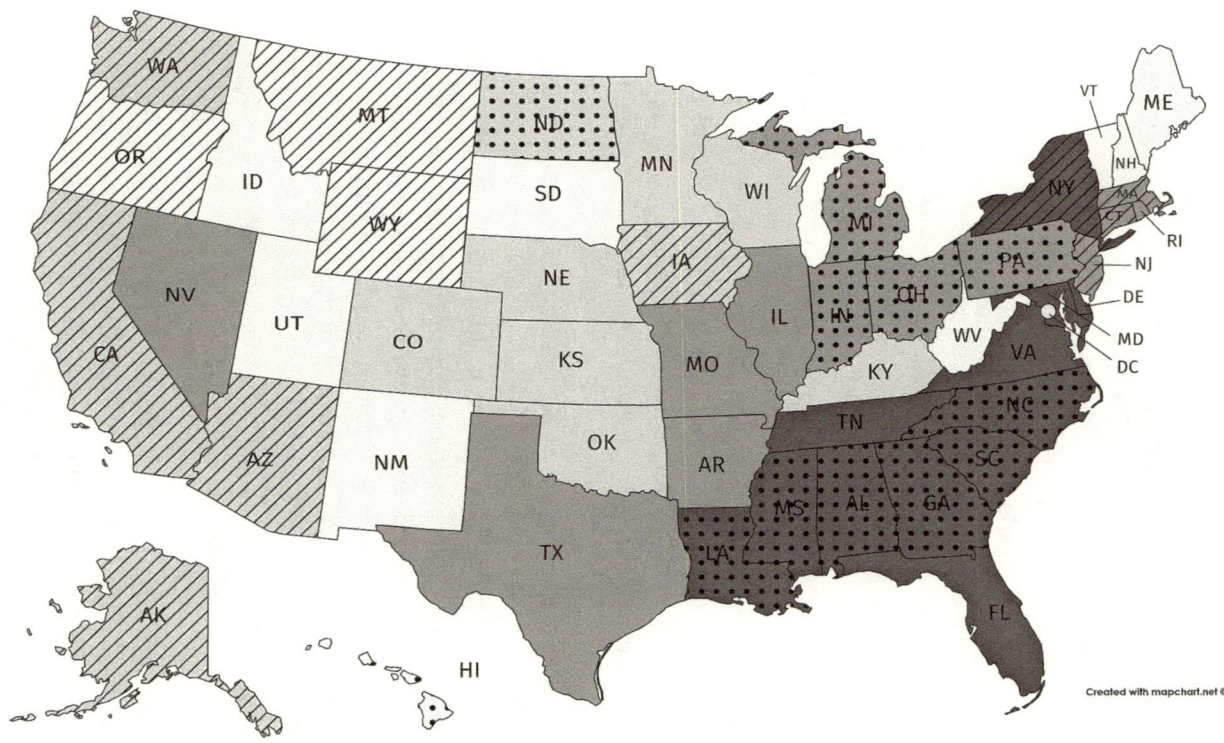

Map B: Percent of Black births per state by quartiles. Deeper shades of gray represent a higher proportion of Black births, and lighter shades represent a lower proportion of Black births. States with diagonal lines show where rates of neonatal mortality are lowest, and states with dots show where rates are highest.

Created with mapchart.net ©

Source: Vedam, S., K. Stoll, M. MacDorman, E. Declercq, R. Cramer, M. Cheyney, T. Fisher, et al. 2018. "Mapping Integration of Midwives across the United States: Impact on Access, Equity, and Outcomes." *PLoS ONE* 13(2): e0192523. https://doi.org/10.1371/journal.pone.0192523.

Evidence-Based Doula Care

In 2012, 6 percent of birthing people said they used a doula during childbirth (Declercq et al. 2013), up from 3 percent in a 2006 national survey (Declercq et al. 2007). In 2017, Bohren et al. published an updated Cochrane review on the use of continuous support for people during childbirth. The birthing people in these studies were randomized to either receive continuous one-on-one support during labor or the "usual care" provided by hospital staff. Overall, people who received continuous support by doulas were 15 percent more likely to have spontaneous vaginal births and less likely to have any pain medication. People who received continual care by doulas were 39 percent less likely to have a cesarean birth. In addition, their labors were shorter, and their babies were less likely to have low Apgar scores at birth. There is some evidence that doula support in labor can lower postpartum depression in mothers. There is *no* evidence for negative consequences to continuous labor support. Access to continuous labor support from a doula is especially vital for birthing people of color, as Black people experience higher rates of poor birth outcomes, including higher rates of cesarean, preterm birth, low birth weight, and infant death (Thomas et al. 2017).

Sources: Declercq, E. R., C. Sakala, M. P. Corry, and S. Applebaum. 2007. "Listening to Mothers II: Report of the Second National U.S. Survey of Women's Childbearing Experiences." *The Journal of Perinatal Education* 16: 9–14; Declercq, E. R., C. Sakala, M. P. Corry, and S. Applebaum. 2013. *Listening to Mothers III Pregnancy and Birth: Report of the Third National*

U.S. Survey of Women's Childbearing Experiences. New York: Childbirth Connection; Thomas, M. P., G. Ammann, E. Brazier, and P. Noyes. 2017. "Doula Services within a Healthy Start Program: Increasing Access for an Underserved Population." *Maternal and Child Health Journal* 21(Suppl 1): 59–64; https://evidencebasedbirth.com/the-evidence-for-doulas/.

Documents

The Sheppard-Towner Act (1921)

The National Maternity and Infancy Protection Act, also called the Sheppard-Towner Act, was passed by Congress in November 1921. The Sheppard-Towner Act provided federal funds to states to establish programs to educate people about prenatal health and infant welfare with the hope of addressing the high infant mortality rates in the United States. The funding provided led to the establishment of nearly 3,000 prenatal care clinics, 180,000 infant care seminars, over 3 million home visits by traveling nurses, and a national distribution of educational literature between 1921 and 1928. Historians note that infant mortality did decrease during the years the act was in effect. Although the act was repealed in 1929, it influenced provisions aimed at infant and maternity welfare in later legislation, such as the Social Security Act of 1935.

An Act for the promotion of the welfare and hygiene of maternity and infancy, and for other purposes.

Be it enacted by the Senate and House of Representatives of the United States of America in Congress assembled, That there is hereby authorized to be appropriated annually, out of any money in the Treasury not otherwise appropriated, the sums specified in section 2 of this Act, to be paid to the several States for the purpose of cooperating with them in promoting the welfare and hygiene of maternity and infancy as hereinafter provided.

Sec. 2. For the purpose of carrying out the provision of this Act, there is authorized to be appropriated, out of any money in the Treasury not otherwise appropriated, for the current fiscal year $480,000, to be equally apportioned among the several States, and for each subsequent year, for the period of five years, $240,000, to be equally apportioned for the use of the States, subject to the provisions of this Act, for the fiscal year ending June 30, 1922, an additional sum of $1,000,000, and annually thereafter, for the period of five years, an additional sum not to exceed $1,000,000. Provided further, That the additional appropriations herein authorized shall be apportioned $5,000 to each State and the balance among the States in the proportion which their population bears to the total population of the States of the United States, according to the last preceding United States census: And provided further, That no payment out of the additional appropriation herein authorized shall be made in any year to any State until an equal sum has been appropriated for that year by the legislature of such State for the maintenance of the services and facilities provided for in this Act.

So much of the amount apportioned to any State for any fiscal year as remains unpaid to such State at the close thereof shall be available for expenditures in that State until the close of the succeeding fiscal year.

Sec. 3. There is hereby created a Board of Maternity and Infant Hygiene, which shall consist of the Chief of the Children's Bureau, the Surgeon General of the United States Public Health Service, and the United States Commissioner of Education, and which is hereafter designated in this Act of the Board. The Board shall elect its own chairman and perform the duties provided for in this Act.

The Children's Bureau of the Department of Labor shall be charged with the administration of this Act, except as herein otherwise provided, and the Chief of the Children's Bureau shall be the executive officer. It shall be the duty of the Children's Bureau to make or cause to be such studies, investigations, and reports as will promote the efficient administration of this Act.

Source: 42 Stat. 224 (Pub. Law 67-97), November 23, 1921.

Childbirth Connection Blueprint for Action (2010)

Founded in 1918 as the Maternity Center Association, Childbirth Connection is now a core program of the National Partnership for Women & Families. Childbirth Connection offers evidence-based birth information through policy and quality initiatives and is focused on transforming the nation's maternity care system so that childbearing women and babies consistently receive high-quality, woman- and family-centered care. In 2008, Childbirth Connection hosted a 90th anniversary national policy symposium, Transforming Maternity Care: A High Value Proposition, on April 3, 2009, in Washington, DC. Over 100 leaders from across the range of stakeholder perspectives were actively engaged in the symposium work to improve the quality and value of U.S. maternity care through broad system improvement and to answer the question, Who needs to do what to, for, and with whom to improve maternity care quality within the next five years?

Childbirth Connection marked its 90th Anniversary with the multi-stakeholder Transforming Maternity Care Symposium, held on April 3, 2009, in Washington, DC. The project began with the development of a direction-setting paper, the "2020 Vision for a High-Quality, High-Value Maternity Care System." It brought together policy makers, public and private purchasers and payors, administrators, advocates, clinicians, educators, researchers, and quality experts to devise feasible solutions to transform the U.S. maternity care system so that it reliably delivers high-quality, high-value care that is optimal for women and babies.

The goal of the Transforming Maternity Care symposium was to answer the question: Who needs to do what, to, for, and with whom to improve maternity care quality within the next 5 years?

More than 100 leading experts contributed to the project, and close to 250 people attended the symposium. Five stakeholder workgroups collaborated to develop reports and recommendations that offer concrete solutions to salient issues. The development of actionable strategies to improve maternity care quality and value centered on 11 critical focus areas for change:

- Performance measurement and leveraging of results
- Payment reform to align incentives with quality
- Disparities in access and outcomes of maternity care
- Improved functioning of the liability system
- Scope of covered services for maternity care
- Coordination of maternity care, across time, settings, and disciplines
- Clinical controversies (home birth, vaginal birth after cesarean [VBAC], vaginal breech and twin birth, elective induction, and cesarean section without indication)
- Decision making and consumer choice
- Scope, content, and availability of health professions education
- Workforce composition and distribution
- Development and use of health information technology (IT).

This Executive Summary presents the major recommendations to come out of the Transforming Maternity Care project at a glance (see below). The main body describes, for each of the critical focus areas: leading concerns with the status quo, system goals, priority recommendations and action steps for their implementation, and the sectors, organizations and agencies with lead responsibilities. The five full stakeholder workgroup reports, which provide in rich detail the sector-specific strategies that gave rise to this comprehensive roadmap for improvement of the U.S. maternity care system, can be accessed online at www.childbirthconnection.org/workgroups.

Source: Angood, P. B., E. M. Armstrong, D. Ashton, H. Burstin, M. P. Corry, S. F. Delbanco, B. Fildes, et al. 2010. "Blueprint for Action Steps Toward a High-Quality, High-Value Maternity Care System." *Women's Health Issues* (January–February).

https://doi.org/10.1016/j.whi.2009.11.007. Reprinted with permission from Elsevier.

Improving Access to Maternity Care Act (2017)

The Improving Access to Maternity Care Act was introduced by Senator Tammy Baldwin (D-WI) and Congressman Michael Burgess (R-TX) in 2017 and became law in 2018. The Improving Access to Maternity Care Act has two main objectives: the first is to require the Health Resources and Services Administration (HRSA) to collect and analyze data to generate information on maternity health professional shortage areas (HPSA), leading to the designation of maternity care shortage areas. The second is to provide maternity care shortage area data to the National Health Service Corps (NHSC) to ensure that maternity care resources are targeted to the areas where they are most needed. The National Health Service Corps provides student loan repayment to physicians and other health professionals in exchange for a commitment by those professionals to provide care in designated HPSAs.

An Act
To amend the Public Health Service Act to distribute maternity care health professionals to health professional shortage areas identified as in need of maternity care health services.

Be it enacted by the Senate and House of Representatives of the United States of America in Congress assembled,

SECTION 1. SHORT TITLE.
This Act may be cited as the "Improving Access to Maternity Care Act."

SEC. 2. MATERNITY CARE HEALTH PROFESSIONAL TARGET AREAS.
Section 332 of the Public Health Service Act (42 U.S.C. 254e) is amended by adding at the end the following new subsection:

"(k)(1) The Secretary, acting through the Administrator of the Health Resources and Services Administration, shall identify, based on the data collected under paragraph (3), maternity care health professional target areas that satisfy the criteria described in paragraph (2) for purposes of, in connection with receipt of assistance under this title, assigning to such identified areas maternity care health professionals who, without application of this subsection, would otherwise be eligible for such assistance. The Secretary shall distribute maternity care health professionals within health professional shortage areas using the maternity care health professional target areas so identified.

(2) For purposes of paragraph (1), the Secretary shall establish criteria for maternity care health professional target areas that identify geographic areas within health professional shortage areas that have a shortage of maternity care health professionals.

(3) For purposes of this subsection, the Secretary shall collect and publish in the Federal Register data comparing the availability and need of maternity care health services in health professional shortage areas and in areas within such health professional shortage areas.

(4) In carrying out paragraph (1), the Secretary shall seek input from relevant provider organizations, including medical societies, organizations representing medical facilities, and other organizations with expertise in maternity care.

(5) For purposes of this subsection, the term 'full scope maternity care health services' includes during labor care, birthing, prenatal care, and postpartum care.

(6) Nothing in this subsection shall be construed as—

(A) requiring the identification of a maternity care health professional target area in an area not otherwise already designated as a health professional shortage area; or

(B) affecting the types of health professionals, without application of this subsection, otherwise eligible for assistance, including a loan repayment or scholarship, pursuant to the application of this section."

Source: 132 Stat. 4438, Public Law 115-320, December 17, 2018. Available online at https://congress.gov/115/plaws /publ320/PLAW-115publ320.pdf.

Black Maternal Health Momnibus Act (2020)

The Black Maternal Health Momnibus Act was first introduced by Representative Lauren Underwood (D-IL) in March of 2020. The Act's stated purpose is to end preventable maternal mortality and severe maternal morbidity in the United States and close disparities in maternal health outcomes. If passed, this will be historical legislation toward addressing social determinants of health and diversifying the perinatal health workforce. Below is one of eight key areas—perinatal workforce—that the Act addresses.

TITLE IV—PERINATAL WORKFORCE

(a) GUIDANCE TO STATES.—

(1) IN GENERAL.—Not later than 2 years after the date of enactment of this Act, the Secretary of Health and Human Services shall issue and disseminate guidance to States to educate providers and managed care entities about the value and process of delivering respectful maternal health care through diverse care provider models.

(2) CONTENTS.—The guidance required by paragraph (1) shall address how States can encourage and incentivize hospitals, health systems, freestanding birth centers, other maternity care provider groups, and managed care entities—

(A) to recruit and retain maternity care providers, such as obstetrician-gynecologists, family physicians, physician assistants, midwives who meet at a minimum the international definition of the midwife and global standards for midwifery education as established by the International Confederation of Midwives, nurse practitioners, and clinical nurse specialists—

(i) from racially and ethnically diverse backgrounds;

(ii) with experience practicing in racially and ethnically diverse communities; and

(iii) who have undergone trainings on implicit and explicit bias and racism;

(B) to incorporate into maternity care teams midwives who meet at a minimum the international definition of the midwife and global standards for midwifery education as established by the International Confederation of Midwives, doulas, community health workers, peer supporters, certified lactation consultants, nutritionists and dietitians, social workers, home visitors, and navigators;

(C) to provide collaborative, culturally congruent care; and

(D) to provide opportunities for individuals enrolled in accredited midwifery education programs to participate in job shadowing with maternity care teams in hospitals, health systems, and freestanding birth centers.

(b) STUDY ON CULTURALLY CONGRUENT MATERNITY CARE.—

(1) STUDY.—The Secretary of Health and Human Services acting through the Director of the National Institutes of Health (in this subsection referred to as the "Secretary") shall conduct a study on best practices in culturally congruent maternity care.

(2) REPORT.—Not later than 2 years after the date of enactment of this Act, the Secretary shall—

(A) complete the study required by paragraph (1);

(B) submit to the Congress and make publicly available a report on the results of such study; and

(C) include in such report—

(i) a compendium of examples of hospitals, health systems, freestanding birth centers, other maternity care provider groups, and managed care entities that are delivering culturally congruent maternal health care;

(ii) a compendium of examples of hospitals, health systems, freestanding birth centers, other maternity care provider groups, and managed care entities that have low levels of racial and ethnic disparities in maternal health outcomes; and

(iii) recommendations to hospitals, health systems, freestanding birth centers, other maternity care provider groups, and managed care entities for best practices in culturally congruent maternity care.

SEC. 402. GRANTS TO GROW AND DIVERSIFY THE PERINATAL WORKFORCE.

Title VII of the Public Health Service Act is amended by inserting after section 757 (42 U.S.C. 294f) the following new section:

"SEC. 758. PERINATAL WORKFORCE GRANTS.

"(a) IN GENERAL.—The Secretary may award grants to entities to establish or expand programs described in subsection (b) to grow and diversify the perinatal workforce.

"(b) USE OF FUNDS.—Recipients of grants under this section shall use the grants to grow and diversify the perinatal workforce by—

"(1) establishing schools or programs that provide education and training to individuals seeking appropriate licensing or certification as—

"(A) physician assistants who will complete clinical training in the field of maternal and perinatal health; and

"(B) other perinatal health workers such as doulas, community health workers, peer supporters, certified lactation consultants, nutritionists and dietitians, social workers, home visitors, and navigators; and

"(2) expanding the capacity of existing schools or programs described in paragraph (1), for the purposes of increasing the number of students enrolled in such schools or programs, including by awarding scholarships for students.

"(c) PRIORITIZATION.—In awarding grants under this section, the Secretary shall give priority to any institution of higher education that—

"(1) has demonstrated a commitment to recruiting and retaining minority students, particularly from demographic groups experiencing high rates of maternal mortality and severe maternal morbidity;

"(2) has developed a strategy to recruit and retain a diverse pool of students into the perinatal workforce program or school supported by funds received through the grant, particularly from demographic groups experiencing high rates of maternal mortality and severe maternal morbidity;

"(3) has developed a strategy to recruit and retain students who plan to practice in a health professional shortage area designated under section 332;

"(4) has developed a strategy to recruit and retain students who plan to practice in an area with significant racial and ethnic disparities in maternal health outcomes; and

"(5) includes in the standard curriculum for all students within the perinatal workforce program or school a bias, racism, or discrimination training program that includes training on explicit and implicit bias.

"(d) REPORTING.—As a condition on receipt of a grant under this section for a perinatal workforce program or school, an entity shall agree to submit to the Secretary an annual report on the activities conducted through the grant, including—

"(1) the number and demographics of students participating in the program or school;

"(2) the extent to which students in the program or school are entering careers in—

"(A) health professional shortage areas designated under section 332; and

"(B) areas with significant racial and ethnic disparities in maternal health outcomes; and

"(3) whether the program or school has included in the standard curriculum for all students a bias, racism, or discrimination training program that includes explicit and implicit bias, and if so the effectiveness of such training program.

"(e) PERIOD OF GRANTS.—The period of a grant under this section shall be up to 5 years.

"(f) APPLICATION.—To seek a grant under this section, an entity shall submit to the Secretary an application at such time, in such manner, and containing such information as the Secretary may require, including any information necessary for prioritization under subsection (c).

"(g) TECHNICAL ASSISTANCE.—The Secretary shall provide, directly or by contract, technical assistance to institutions of higher education seeking or receiving a grant under this section on the development, use, evaluation, and post-grant period sustainability of the perinatal workforce programs or schools proposed to be, or being, established or expanded through the grant.

"(h) REPORT BY SECRETARY.—Not later than 4 years after the date of enactment of this section, the Secretary shall prepare and submit to the Congress, and post on the internet website of the Department of Health and Human Services, a report on the effectiveness of the grant program under this section at—

"(1) recruiting minority students, particularly from demographic groups experiencing high rates of maternal mortality and severe maternal morbidity;

"(2) increasing the number of physician assistants who will complete clinical training in the field of maternal and perinatal health, and other perinatal health workers, from demographic groups experiencing high rates of maternal mortality and severe maternal morbidity;

"(3) increasing the number of physician assistants who will complete clinical training in the field of maternal and perinatal health, and other perinatal health workers, working in health professional shortage areas designated under section 332; and

"(4) increasing the number of physician assistants who will complete clinical training in the field of maternal and perinatal health, and other perinatal health workers, working in areas with significant racial and ethnic disparities in maternal health outcomes.

"(i) AUTHORIZATION OF APPROPRIATIONS.—To carry out this section, there is authorized to be appropriated $15,000,000 for each of fiscal years 2021 through 2025."

SEC. 403. GRANTS TO GROW AND DIVERSIFY THE NURSING WORKFORCE IN MATERNAL AND PERINATAL HEALTH.

Title VIII of the Public Health Service Act is amended by inserting after section 811 of that Act (42 U.S.C. 296j) the following:

"SEC. 812. PERINATAL NURSING WORKFORCE GRANTS.

"(a) In General.—The Secretary may award grants to schools of nursing to grow and diversify the perinatal nursing workforce.

"(b) Use Of Funds.—Recipients of grants under this section shall use the grants to grow and diversify the perinatal nursing workforce by providing scholarships to students seeking to become—

"(1) nurse practitioners whose education includes a focus on maternal and perinatal health; or

"(2) clinical nurse specialists whose education includes a focus on maternal and perinatal health.

"(c) Prioritization.—In awarding grants under this section, the Secretary shall give priority to any school of nursing that—

"(1) has developed a strategy to recruit and retain a diverse pool of students seeking to enter careers focused on maternal and perinatal health;

"(2) has developed a partnership with a practice setting in a health professional shortage area designated under section 332 for the clinical placements of the school's students;

"(3) has developed a strategy to recruit and retain students who plan to practice in an area with significant racial and ethnic disparities in maternal health outcomes; and

"(4) includes in the standard curriculum for all students seeking to enter careers focused on maternal and perinatal health a bias, racism, or discrimination training program that includes education on explicit and implicit bias.

"(d) Reporting.—As a condition on receipt of a grant under this section, a school of nursing shall agree to submit to the Secretary an annual report on the activities conducted through the grant, including, to the extent practicable—

"(1) the number and demographics of students in the school of nursing seeking to enter careers focused on maternal and perinatal health;

"(2) the extent to which such students are preparing to enter careers in—

"(A) health professional shortage areas designated under section 332; and

"(B) areas with significant racial and ethnic disparities in maternal health outcomes; and

"(3) whether the standard curriculum for all students seeking to enter careers focused on maternal and perinatal health includes a bias, racism, or discrimination training program that includes education on explicit and implicit bias.

"(e) PERIOD OF GRANTS.—The period of a grant under this section shall be up to 5 years.

"(f) APPLICATION.—To seek a grant under this section, an entity shall submit to the Secretary an application, at such time, in such manner, and containing such information as the Secretary may require, including any information necessary for prioritization under subsection (c).

"(g) TECHNICAL ASSISTANCE.—The Secretary shall provide, directly or by contract, technical assistance to schools of nursing seeking or receiving a grant under this section on the processes of awarding and evaluating scholarships through the grant.

"(h) REPORT BY SECRETARY.—Not later than 4 years after the date of enactment of this section, the Secretary shall prepare and submit to the Congress, and post on the internet website of the Department of Health and Human Services, a report on the effectiveness of the grant program under this section at—

"(1) recruiting minority students, particularly from demographic groups experiencing high rates of maternal mortality and severe maternal morbidity;

"(2) increasing the number of nurse practitioners and clinical nurse specialists entering careers focused on maternal and perinatal health from demographic groups experiencing high rates of maternal mortality and severe maternal morbidity;

"(3) increasing the number of nurse practitioners and clinical nurse specialists entering careers focused on maternal and perinatal health working in health professional shortage areas designated under section 332; and

"(4) increasing the number of nurse practitioners and clinical nurse specialists entering careers focused on maternal and perinatal health working in areas with significant racial and ethnic disparities in maternal health outcomes.

"(i) AUTHORIZATION OF APPROPRIATIONS.—To carry out this section, there is authorized to be appropriated $15,000,000 for each of fiscal years 2021 through 2025."

SEC. 404. GAO REPORT ON BARRIERS TO MATERNITY CARE.

(a) IN GENERAL.—Not later than two years after the date of the enactment of this Act and every five years thereafter, the Comptroller General of the United States shall submit to Congress a report on barriers to maternity care in the United States. Such report shall include the information and recommendations described in subsection (b).

(b) CONTENT OF REPORT.—The report under subsection (a) shall include—

(1) an assessment of current barriers to entering accredited midwifery education programs, and recommendations for addressing such barriers, particularly for low-income and minority women;

(2) an assessment of current barriers to entering accredited education programs for other maternity care professional careers, including obstetrician-gynecologists, family physicians, physician assistants, nurse practitioners, and clinical nurse specialists, particularly for low-income and minority women;

(3) an assessment of current barriers that prevent midwives from meeting the international definition of the midwife and global standards for midwifery education as established by the International Confederation of Midwives, and recommendations for addressing such barriers, particularly for low-income and minority women; and

(4) recommendations to promote greater equity in compensation for perinatal health workers, particularly for such individuals from racially and ethnically diverse backgrounds.

Source: H.R.6142 – Black Maternal Health Momnibus Act of 2020.https://www.congress.gov/bill/116th-congress/house-bill/6142/text#toc-H5E605AC1178F48CDBF60CCA1E20A3216.

Organizational Commitments to Equity

Health care providers must be representative of the nation's population. It is imperative for professional organizations to actively commit to recruiting, retaining, and supporting diverse providers in terms of race-ethnicity, gender identity and expression, sexual orientation, religion, and so on. Diverse providers are essential to health equity. The following documents are the commitments to equity made by the National Association of Certified Professional Midwives and the American College of Nurse-Midwives.

National Association of Certified Professional Midwives

We know that quality maternity care is presently not the norm for most women in the U.S. Our over-use of expensive technologies and underuse of many beneficial forms of care has resulted in the most expensive maternity health care system in the world with relatively poor outcomes: our perinatal, infant and maternal mortality rates are worse than almost all other wealthy nations, and even worse than many poorer nations who spend far less that we do. Against this backdrop, the outcomes of mothers and babies of color are shockingly disparate. Black mothers are 4 times more likely to die of pregnancy-related complications than their white counterparts, and their babies are 2.5 times more likely to die in their first year of life. American Indians and Alaska Natives have an infant death rate 60 percent higher than the rate for whites. Although a key cause of these disparities may be unequal access to quality care, we recognize that societal and institutional racism, a system of power based on color, is the root cause.

Undoing societal and institutional racism in all its forms and eliminating maternity care disparities in our country is an enormous task. There can be no quick fixes. NACPM recognizes that we must make a commitment to doing work in our own sphere: that of strengthening our professional association of CPMs in service of improving the maternity care system in the U.S., and of supporting the work of other stakeholders within their spheres of influence and partnering with them to make a difference.

Towards this end, the Board of Directors and Staff of NACPM intend to work in the following ways to address institutional racism personally and in our profession and to work more effectively to eliminate racial disparities in the health of mothers and babies in the U.S.:

1. We commit to addressing racism on an individual, board, and organizational level.

    - Each board and staff member commits to pursuing personal anti-racism training.
    - The board and staff commit to regular study-discussion together during board conference calls and in-face board meetings.
    - We acknowledge and appreciate the work of the Anti-Racism and Anti-Oppression Work in Midwifery group that emerged from the CPM Symposium 2012, and will encourage NACPM members to participate and access the anti-racism training resources this group provides. Follow their blog. Join the conversation on Facebook.

2. We desire and require the leadership of people of color as board members and advisors to the board in all aspects of the work of the organization.

    - Because of the urgency of including people of color in key leadership positions in NACPM, and in direct response to a request made by people of color at the CPM Symposium, the Board has expanded the number of board members from 5 to 8 and appointed two midwives of color to fill these positions.

3. The Board will reach out to experts for assistance in developing a multi-disciplinary Advisory Group on Maternity Care Disparities to advise the NACPM board and staff so that our professional association can work more effectively and partner with other groups and organizations to address racial disparities in maternity care.

4. We recognize that it is urgent to increase the number of midwives of color in the U.S. and that significant barriers to midwifery education exist for people of color. We commit to partnering with other organizations and individuals to address barriers and challenges and expand access to education.

5. We recognize cultural sensitivity, versatility, and safety to be core competencies in midwifery care and will support, influence, and align with the work of partner organizations to move forward in incorporating these requirements into midwifery education and practice standards.

6. We commit to the continuation of our policy work to expand access for all women to the care of CPMs, which at its heart addresses key components to equal access to care, and must include the leadership and expertise of people of color.

Source: https://nacpm.org/for-cpms/social-justice/strategic -intention/. Used by permission.

American College of Nurse-Midwives

"Shifting the Frame" highlights the strengths and positive values midwives can draw on to improve our ability to work in a multicultural world. And it also challenges us to do more to actively listen and learn about ourselves and others who have had different lived experiences. To all midwives whose lives have been touched by injustice and inequity, we honor you and extend our compassion. This report urges us to do more to support you and to create a more just and equitable society.

Some parts of the report are difficult to read—for example, when we read about how ACNM has previously fallen short in meeting the needs of midwives of color. Also, the report discusses concepts that are outside of our typical work as midwives and may take time and learning to fully understand. We've provided additional learning resources along with the report which we hope you will take time to explore.

"Shifting the Frame" tells us clearly that ACNM needs to be a more open, accessible organization for all members and provide leadership opportunities for everyone. We have grown well beyond the small circle of midwives who initially made ACNM possible in 1955. With double digit growth in our profession, and the most diverse and dynamic US population in history, it's time for us to re-envision the future of our organization and our profession. This focus will enhance the professional lives of all of our members, and especially those from traditionally underrepresented groups.

It has our strong desire and intention to be an organization that provides equal opportunities for active participation and leadership for all members. We are fully dedicated to identifying and breaking down barriers to this vision, as we believe that our ability to transform women's health for the better depends on our success. It's time to put our desires and vision into action.

Source: "Shifting the Frame," © 2015 Jodi DeLibertis/American College of Nurse-Midwives. Used by permission.

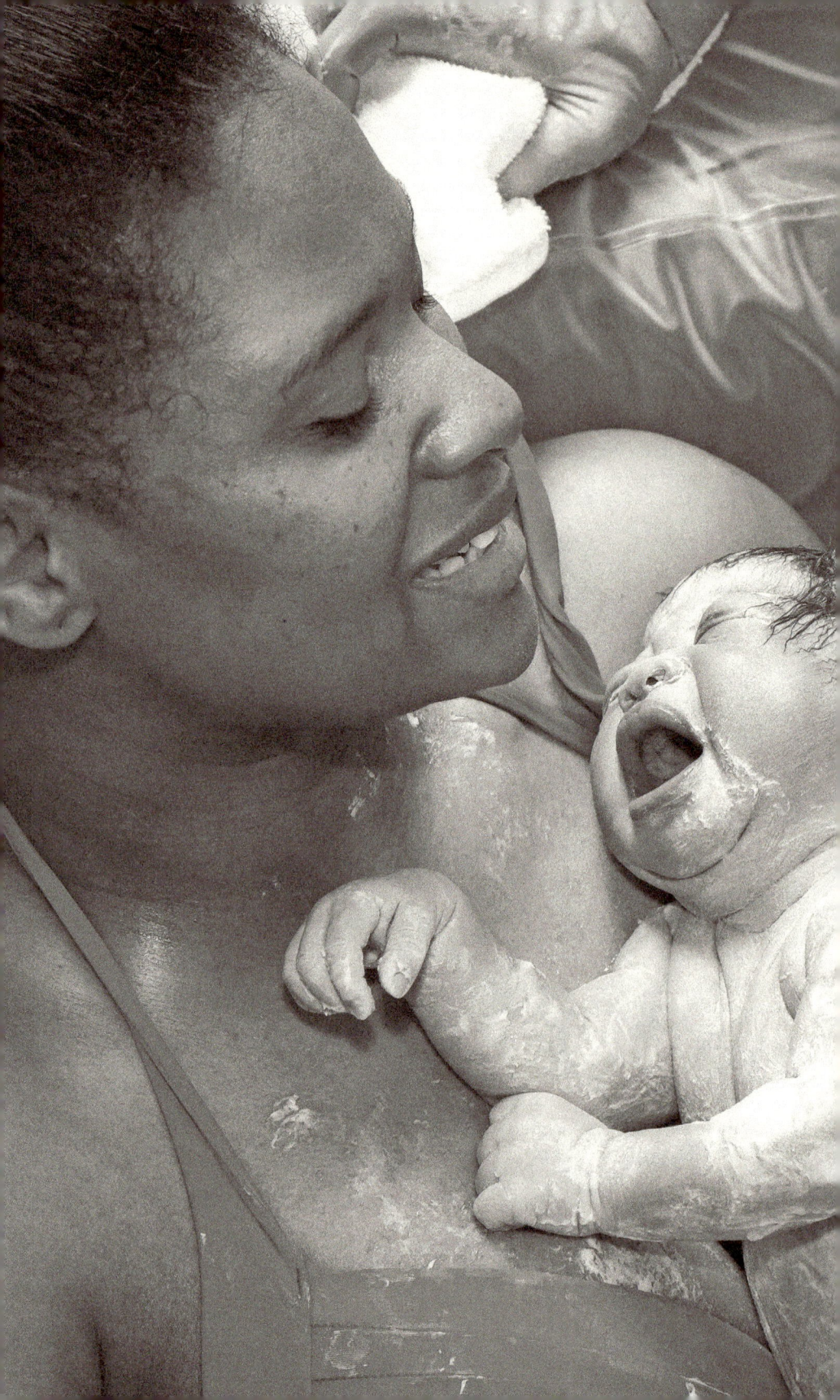

This chapter provides the reader with next steps for research on the topics of pregnancy and birth in the United States. In this annotated bibliography, the reader will find material on the medicalization of pregnancy and birth; assisted reproductive technology and surrogacy; media representations of pregnancy and birth; racial and ethnic birth disparities and inequities; and, experiences of pregnant and birthing LGBTQ people and families.

Much has been written and produced on the topic of pregnancy and birth in the United States. This chapter is not intended to represent a comprehensive authority on the subject, but rather to include a sampling of work to introduce the reader into further research. Materials included are books, articles, journals, websites, podcasts, film, television, and digital media.

Books

Addison, H., M. K. Goodwin-Kelly, and E. Roth, eds. 2009. *Motherhood Misconceived: Representing the Maternal in U.S. Films*. Albany: State University New York Press.

    This book is an anthology of essays that explore motherhood and pregnancy as portrayed in mainstream and independent cinema.

A water birth. (Jbrown777/Dreamstime.com)

Apfel, A. 2016. *Birth Work as Care Work: Stories from Activist Birth Communities*. Oakland, CA: PM Press.
> This book presents a vibrant collection of stories and insights from the perspective of birth activist communities.

Armstrong, P., and S. Feldman. 1986. *A Midwife's Story*. New York: Arbor House.
> This book is a biographical account of the author's transition from student midwife in Glasgow to working among the Old Order Amish in Lancaster, Pennsylvania. This narrative recounts the author's experience about learning about natural birth from the Amish community.

Ashford, J. I. 1998. *Natural Love: A Parody*. Solana Beach, CA: J. Ashford.
> This book is a science fiction parody that looks at the relationship between childbirth and technology. The narrative explores what it would be like to make love in a hospital under the same medicalized technology that childbirth is subjected to in hospitals today.

Barber, K. 2005. *The Black Woman's Guide to Breastfeeding: The Definitive Guide to Nursing for African American Mothers*. Chicago: Sourcebooks, Incorporated.
> This book is an instructional manual for African American mothers on the subject of breastfeeding.

Beatie, T. 2008. *Labor of Love: The Story of One Man's Extraordinary Pregnancy*. Berkeley, CA: Seal Press.
> This is an autobiographical account of Thomas Beatie. Beatie is a transman whose pregnancy in 2008 became international news. This is a very intimate look at the author's life, pregnancy, family, and identity.

Block, J. 2008. *Pushed: The Painful Truth about Childbirth and Modern Maternity Care.* Cambridge, MA: Da Capo.

This book takes an investigative journalist's look at modern childbirth in the United States and reveals the uncomfortable truths about the use of routine interventions in medical birth management. The author shows the role between the high rates of medical interventions with the high cesarean rates and high infant and maternal mortality rates in the United States. Block places the routine interventions used in American maternity care within a complex matrix of medical institutional finance needs and liability, provider licensing, and regulation interests and shows that these interventions often have little to do with the evidence-based needs of birthing people.

Bohjalian, C. 1998. *Midwives: A Novel.* New York: Vintage Books.

In this work of fiction, the storyline follows a rural midwife in Vermont who is accused of killing one of her patients by the deceased patient's husband. This work is one of the first to represent community midwives.

Bovard, W. L., and G. Milton. 1993. *Why Not Me? The Story of Gladys Milton, Midwife.* Summertown, TN: Book Publishing Company.

This book is a biography of Gladys Milton, written by Gladys Milton and her friend Wendy Bovard. Gladys Milton had a long career as a licensed midwife in the state of Florida. She was an advocate of women's health and traditional midwifery and provided care to women in rural Florida. The narrative retells the story of her life, her profession, and her fight against the Florida Health Department when it tried to revoke her midwifery license and force her to retire.

Bridges, K. M. 2011. *Reproducing Race: An Ethnography of Pregnancy as a Site of Racialization*. Berkeley: University of California Press.
This book is an ethnography of pregnancy and birth at a large New York City hospital. The author explores how the social construction of race and class impacts pregnant and birthing people in hospital settings.

Briggs, L. 2018. *How All Politics Became Reproductive Politics: From Welfare Reform to Foreclosure to Trump*. Oakland: University of California Press.
This book argues that all politics are reproductive politics, and between longer work hours and the election of President Donald Trump, the current political crisis is centered around reproductive rights.

Brill, S. 2006. *The New Essential Guide to Lesbian Conception, Pregnancy & Birth*. New York: Alyson.
This book is an educational resource for lesbians and all families looking to achieve pregnancy via donor insemination. While this book is an excellent resource for families wanting to get pregnant, it is also a great resource for care providers who want to provide more culturally appropriate care for their lesbian clients.

Buss, F. L. 1980. *La Partera: Story of a Midwife*. Ann Arbor: University of Michigan Press.
This is the biographical tale of Jesusita Aragon, a midwife who practiced in New Mexico. Jesusita was trained by her grandmother in traditional Hispanic midwifery practices, and she delivered over 12,000 babies to rural women in New Mexico over the span of her career.

Carsten, J. 2003. *After Kinship*. Cambridge, UK: Cambridge University Press.
This book looks at the anthropological study of kinship and the future of the study of kinship. The author asks questions about the impact of reproductive technologies,

changing ideas about gender, and the social construction of science on the study of kinship.

Conrad, P. 2007. *The Medicalization of Society: On the Transformation of Human Conditions into Treatable Disorders*. Baltimore: Johns Hopkins University Press.
The author explores the changing forces behind normal human events such as birth, aging, menopause, alcoholism, and obesity becoming medical conditions. The emergence of and changes in medicalization, consequences of expanding the medical domain, and implications for health and society are also examined.

Corea, G. 1988. *The Mother Machine: Reproductive Technologies from Artificial Insemination to Artificial Wombs*. London: Women's Press.
In this book, the author looks at questions about the then new reproductive technologies and their political and social impact on people's lives. The author interviewed research scientists, physicians, patients, ethicists, attorneys, and business executives who work with reproductive technologies, including in vitro fertilization, embryo transfer, artificial insemination, sex predetermination, and the artificial womb.

Davis, D.-A. 2019. *Reproductive Injustice: Racism, Pregnancy, and Premature Birth*. Anthropologies of American Medicine: Culture, Power, and Practice. New York: NYU Press.
This book looks at a troubling study of the role that medical racism plays in the lives of Black women who have given birth to premature and low birth weight infants. Her concept of "obstetric racism," introduced in this book, has been influential to birth and Reproductive Justice providers and researchers.

Davis-Floyd, R., and J. Dumit. 1998. *Cyborg Babies: From Techno-Sex to Techno-Tots*. New York: Routledge.
This book is a collection of essays that examine the relationship between reproductive technologies and the

"cyborgification" of contemporary children. The authors ask questions about the relationship between technoculture and children's emerging consciousness and examine it through science fiction, personal narratives, ethnographic analysis, and social critiques.

Edwards, J., S. Franklin, E. Hirsch, F. Price, and M. Strathern. 1993. *Technologies of Procreation: Kinship in the Age of Assisted Conception*. Manchester, UK: Manchester University Press.
This book looks at the social and cultural implications of reproductive technologies, especially in the context of kinship, from an anthropological perspective.

Ehrenreich, B., and D. English. 2010. *Witches, Midwives, and Nurses: A History of Women Healers*. 2nd ed. New York: Feminist Press.
The original edition of this book was written in 1973 during the second feminist wave. The authors trace the history of women healers and look at the persecution they faced from the institution of medicine.

Ehrensaft, D. 2011. *Mommies, Daddies, Donors, Surrogates: Answering Tough Questions and Building Strong Families*. New York: Guilford Publications.
The author of this book is a clinical psychologist who has helped many families who used reproductive technologies to process their experience. The author brings up many questions that may arise for families after using assisted reproductive technologies and offers insights and advice for dealing with the answers.

Fett, S. 2002. *Working Cures: Healing, Health, and Power on Southern Slave Plantations*. Chapel Hill: University of North Carolina Press.
In this book, the author takes a meaning-centered and critical social and political analysis of the history of enslaved African American health and healing traditions

in the South. The author explores healing, midwifery, herbalism, and conjuring and shows how African American healing arts were acts of resistance to slavery, white supremacy, and white biomedicine. The author frames African American healing within a broad sociopolitical context that explores the relationship between hierarchies of power and healing traditions as well as the culture and community building aspects of healing practices.

Franklin, S., and H. Ragoné. 1998. *Reproducing Reproduction: Kinship, Power, and Technological Innovation.* Philadelphia: University of Pennsylvania Press.

This book looks at the social and cultural aspects of reproduction. The collection of essays uses ethnographic studies and anthropological theory to argue for a new centering of reproductive politics within a political and historical context. Chapters explore topics such as "Obstetrical Ultrasound in American Culture" and "Pregnant Women's Attitudes on Disability within the Context of Prenatal Testing."

Fraser, G. 1998. *African American Midwifery in the South: Dialogues of Birth, Race and Memory.* Cambridge, MA: Harvard University Press.

The author examines how the state and the medical industry worked to bring midwives under supervision and then elimination from practice. This book counters the narrative that the disappearance of African American midwives was inevitable because of medical science progress and professionalization and shows that the disappearance of the midwives was a strategic affront. Through ethnographic analysis and interviews, the book reveals many discourses on midwifery, birth, and race in the southern United States. Parts 1 and 2 of the book focus on the transition of regulation and surveillance, and part 3 focuses on the narratives collected from interviews the author conducted among individuals who remember the African American midwives.

Gaskin, I. M. 1977. *Spiritual Midwifery*. Rev. ed. Summertown, TN: Book Publishing Company.

Originally published in 1977, *Spiritual Midwifery* is now in its fourth edition. The book is considered a classic text from the emerging home birth movement of the 1970s, as it introduced a new generation to home birth and midwifery. The book includes stories of home births as well as a technical manual for midwives. Ina May Gaskin has had a long career in midwifery and is the founder of the Farm Midwifery Center.

Golden, J. 2001. *A Social History of Wet Nursing in America: From Breast to Bottle*. Columbus: Ohio State University Press.

In this book, the author looks at how social constructions of motherhood, medical science, class, race and culture intersect in the history of wet nursing from the colonial period to the twentieth-century United States.

Gonzales, P. 2015. *Red Medicine: Traditional Indigenous Rites of Birthing and Healing*. Tucson: University of Arizona Press.

The author explores Indigenous healing practices across North America, with particular focus on Mexico. Patrisia Gonzales is a scholar, herbalist, and traditional birth attendant and includes her own personal experiences with storytelling and oral tradition research, symbolic interpretation, elder knowledge, and Indigenous research. The book pays particular attention to Spiderwoman knowledge.

Jordan, B. 1978. *Birth in Four Cultures: A Cross Cultural Investigation of Childbirth in Yucatan, Holland, Sweden, and the United States*. Long Grove, IL: Waveland Press, Inc.

This book is a comparative study of birth based on Brigitte Jordan's fieldwork. The author examines childbirth through different birthing systems. Jordan's work argues against romanticizing traditional cultures' birth practices as less complicated, and she argues that childbirth is a life-altering event in all societies. Jordan received the Margaret Mead Award in recognition of *Birth in Four Cultures.*

Kitzinger, S. 2003. *The Complete Book of Pregnancy and Childbirth.* New York: Alfred A. Knopf.
This book reflects scientific advances and cultural trends in all the information expectant parents need to make their own decisions about everything—from which tests to allow to how to handle pain to where to give birth.

Leavitt, J. W. 1986. *Brought to Bed: Childbearing in America 1750 to 1950.* New York: Oxford University Press.
This book looks at the history of childbirth from colonial times to the late twentieth century. Using personal narratives, the author weaves a history of shifting power from women and home-centered birthing practices to male-controlled medicine and the eventual move of birth to the hospital.

Leavitt, J. W. 2009. *Make Room for Daddy: The Journey from Waiting Room to Birthing Room.* Chapel Hill: University of North Carolina Press.
In this book, historian Judith Walzer Leavitt looks at men's changing roles as fathers and birth attendants in the twentieth century. Leavitt maps out a time frame of five decades, 1935–1985, in which men made their entrance into the birthing rooms. Beginning with the medicalization of birth and ending with men and women together in the birth and delivery rooms, the author provides a history of men's changing relationship to childbirth and to the wider historical narrative of childbirth.

Lee, V. 1996. *Granny Midwives and Black Women Writers: Double-Dutched Readings.* New York: Routledge.
In this history of midwifery, the author takes a unique perspective that she named "double-dutched reading," She contrasts the biographies of historical Black "granny"

midwives and the fiction of Black women writers to show how fiction impacts history and history impacts fiction. This is a unique literary and historical analysis of the granny figure in Black women's midwifery culture.

Logan, O. L., and K. Clark. 1991. *Motherwit: An Alabama Midwife's Story*. New York: Penguin Books.
This book is the biography of midwife Onnie Lee Logan as told to Katherine Clark. Onnie Lee Logan was a Black midwife supporting poor families in rural Alabama for over 40 years. Even after she was forced to give up her license to practice midwifery by the state, she continued on supporting families and providing access to birth care.

MacDonald, T. 2016. *Where's the Mother? Stories from a Transgender Dad*. Winnipeg: Trans Canada Press.
This book explores what it is like to get pregnant, give birth, and breastfeed a child while being an out transgender man, during a time when "pregnancy" is automatically thought of as "motherhood."

Mahoney, M. 2016. *Doulas: Radical Care for Pregnant People*. New York: Feminist Press at the City University of New York.
This book discusses how full-spectrum doulas remain focused on life's physically intimate relationships, such as between caregivers and patients, parents and pregnancy, and individuals and their bodies, while feminism continues to migrate online.

Mamo, L. 2007. *Queering Reproduction: Achieving Pregnancy in the Age of Technoscience*. Durham, NC: Duke University Press.
This book looks at how fertility treatments, such as in vitro fertilization (IVF), have added new options beyond donor insemination for lesbians wanting to have children. It looks at how the reproductive technologies have shifted

the experience of reproduction into a highly medicalized experience and how that shift is affecting the lives and families of lesbians in the United States.

Markens, S. 2007. *Surrogate Motherhood and the Politics of Reproduction*. Berkeley: University of California Press.
This book is an analysis of laws and policy responding to surrogate motherhood in the states of New York and California. The author takes a comprehensive look at the discussions and "culture wars" that are shaping the policy response to surrogacy.

Martens, C., A. P. Gumbs, M. Williams, and J. Jordan. 2016. *Revolutionary Mothering: Love on the Front Lines*. Toronto: Between the Lines.
This anthology is a collection of essays that were written by queer women of color feminists. The essays build on the legacy of the 1960s and 1970s Black and queer feminist work, Reproductive Justice, and more to create a radical manifesto of an anti-racist, anti-capitalist, and anti-oppressive examination of motherhood.

McKay, A. 2006. *The Birth House: A Novel*. 1st U.S. ed. New York: William Morrow.
In this novel, the author spins a narrative about two country midwives in the mid-twentieth century in Canada. The author writes about the challenges they come up against, including the arrival of the male physician who wishes to intervene into their birth practice.

Mitford, J. 1992. *The American Way of Birth*. New York: Dutton.
This book is an investigative look into American birthing practices. The author conducts interviews with obstetricians, midwives, and mothers. She also looks into the surgical, medicalized procedures common in the United

States and examines such issues as the high rates of maternal and infant morbidity in the United States.

Nelson, J. 2003. *Women of Color and the Reproductive Rights Movement*. New York: New York University Press.

This book is a history of women of color in the 1960s and 1970s. The author shows how women of color had distinct reproductive rights issues that were broader than white second-wave feminists' focus on abortion rights. This book takes a look at how feminism, Black nationalism, race, class, and sexuality all intersect within the reproductive rights movement.

Nzinga-Johnson, S. 2013. *Laboring Positions: Black Women, Mothering and the Academy*. Bradford, ON: Demeter Press.

Written by Black women working within academia, this book is an exploration of Black women's lives as mothers and academics. The editor curates a complex and nuanced anthology that examines the intersections of race, gender, mothering, academia, work, and more. Chapters include "Community Property: Black Mother's Communal Ownership of Their Daughters' Degrees" and "Teaching for Change: Notes from a Broke Queer Hustling Mama."

Oparah, J. C., H. Arega, D. Hudson, L. Jones, and T. Oseguera. 2018. *Battling over Birth: Black Women and the Maternal Health Care Crisis*. Amarillo, TX: Praeclarus Press.

This book from the Black Women Birthing Justice Collective is a report that records the experiences of over 100 women who gave birth in California. It looks at how state violence happens in the perinatal health care system for Black women. This book positions Black women's pregnancy and birthing experiences within a human rights framework. It also offers recommendations, solutions, and best practices for holding institutions accountable and improving maternity outcomes for Black women.

Oparah, J. C., and A. D. Bonaparte. 2016. *Birthing Justice: Black Women, Pregnancy, and Childbirth*. New York: Routledge. This book is an anthology of essays exploring Black women's struggle for birth justice. Pulling from a diverse group of authors, including writer/activist Loretta Ross, this book tells many stories of Black women and trans people's experiences in birth and pregnancy. The book is from the Black Women Birthing Justice Collective: http://www .Blackwomenbirthingjustice.org/.

Owens, D. B. C. 2017. *Medical Bondage: Race, Gender, and the Origins of American Gynecology*. Athens: University of Georgia Press. This book is a precise historical investigation of the atrocities committed by nineteenth-century gynecologists—experimental caesarean sections, ovariotomies, and obstetric fistula repairs—on enslaved and poor women. This book examines scientific literature and other communications to expose the advance of obstetrics gained by the dehumanization of vulnerable, disenfranchised people.

Rapp, R. 2000. *Testing Women, Testing the Fetus: The Social Impact of Amniocentesis in America*. New York: Routledge. In this book, the author looks at amniocentesis, a prenatal diagnostic technology, and the social impact and cultural implications of prenatal testing from an anthropological and feminist perspective. The author conducted research for over 15 years, interviewing women and providers from a variety of backgrounds to provide a rich and compelling look into how genetic testing is changing the way we experience pregnancy and birth.

Roberts, D. 1997. *Killing the Black Body: Race, Reproduction and the Meaning of Liberty*. New York: Vintage Books. This book is a an expose on the historical regulation and oppression of Black women's bodies and reproductive rights in the United States, from slavery to the present policies, ideologies, and laws that police and punish Black women's bodies, reproduction, and motherhood. The author shows how the historical oppression and systemic assault of Black women's bodies is and has been central to the construction of the meaning of reproductive freedom in the United States. This book is a classic text in the canon of Reproductive Justice literature.

Roberts, D. 2011. *Fatal Invention: How Science, Politics, and Big Business Re-Create Race in the Twenty-First Century*. New York: New Press.

This groundbreaking book examines how the myth of the biological concept of race—revived by purportedly cutting-edge science, race-specific drugs, genetic testing, and DNA databases—continues to undermine a just society and promote inequality in a supposedly post-racial era. This is essential foundational reading for greater understanding of deeply entrenched racial inequities in pregnancy and childbirth in the United States.

Rooks, J. 1997. *Midwifery and Childbirth in America*. Philadelphia: Temple University Press.

This book is an overview of the history of midwifery and maternity and infant health care in the United States and focuses on the years between 1980 and 1995. The author introduces the reader to the Midwives Model of Care, analyzes the current state of maternal and midwifery care, and provides suggestions for improvement. Specific attention is given to the beginnings of nurse-midwifery, the reproductive rights movements of the 1960s and 1970s, and analyses of research on birth and pregnancy in the United States. The book also examines midwifery models in other industrialized countries.

Ross, L. J., L. Roberts, E. Derkas, W. Peoples, P. Bridgewater Toure, and D. Roberts. 2017. *Radical Reproductive Justice: Foundation, Theory, Practice, Critique*. New York: Feminist Press.
This book is an anthology of essays written by the activists and allies of the SisterSong Women of Color Reproductive Justice Collective. The collection brings together historical, contemporary, and future perspectives on the Reproductive Justice movement. Arranged in four sections, "Historical Context," "Theory," "Policy Practice and Activism," and "Poetry," this book builds on two decades of work and development in the Reproductive Justice movement.

Ross, L. J., and R. Solinger. 2017. *Reproductive Justice: An Introduction*. Oakland: University of California Press.
This book provides a comprehensive description of Reproductive Justice and introduces students to an intersectional analysis of race, class, and gender politics. This book is a classic text in the canon of Reproductive Justice literature.

Rothman, B. Katz. 1982. *In Labor: Women and Power in the Birthplace*. 1st ed. New York: Norton.
This book was the first feminist sociological examination of birth in the United States. The author coined the term "midwifery model" of care and developed a theoretical framework for understanding the two contradicting maternity models of care existing in the United States; the "medical model" and the "midwifery model" of maternity care. The author introduces the reader to the history of obstetrics and shows how U.S. maternity care became male dominated, highly medicalized, and centered in the hospital and compares it with the person-centered approach of midwifery care, where pregnancy is seen as a normal and healthy state of being and people give birth at home attended by midwives.

Rothman, B. Katz. 1989. *Recreating Motherhood: Ideology and Technology in a Patriarchal Society.* 1st ed. New York: Norton.
This book is a social critique of the ideologies that shape motherhood in the United States. In this book, the author argues that conventional ideologies framing motherhood and reproduction—patriarchy, capitalism, and technology—are detrimental to women and children. The author then goes on to offer feminist social alternatives. Part 1 focuses on motherhood under the three ideologies, and part 2 focuses on the possible alternatives.

Rothman, B. Katz. 2016. *A Bun in the Oven: How the Food and Birth Movement Resist Industrialization.* New York: New York University Press.
This book is a comparative historical look at two social movements throughout the twentieth century—the food movement and the birth movement. The author compares the phases of both social movements and how they resist industrialization and strive for meaning and health in food and birth.

Seals-Allers, K. 2017. *The Big Letdown: How Medicine, Big Business, and Feminism Undermine Breastfeeding.* New York: St. Martin's Press.
This book examines the historical, social, and political contexts of American breastfeeding culture and builds a big picture analysis of the structures that shape American women's breastfeeding experiences. The author argues that breastfeeding is not an individual problem, as it is often treated in the U.S. cultural narrative, but a larger social issue shaped by capitalism, the infant formula industry and even an unexpected backlash from feminism.

Simkin, P., and P. H. Klaus. 2011. *When Survivors Give Birth: Understanding and Healing the Effects of Early Sexual Abuse on Childbearing Women.* Seattle: Classic Day Publishing.
This book is written for pregnant people who have experienced childhood sexual abuse and the people who are

their caregivers. The first section is an overview of the effects of sexual abuse on childbearing people. The second section focuses on communication for providers and self-help techniques, and the third section presents clinical challenges and solutions.

Simkin, P., and K. Rohs. 2018. *The Birth Partner: A Complete Guide to Childbirth for Dads, Doulas, and All Other Labor Companions.* Beverly, MA: Harvard Common Press.

The Birth Partner is a comprehensive reference manual for supporting people through labor and the early postpartum period. This book walks the reader through preparing for labor, normal variations and challenges in labor, comfort measures, possible interventions, complications in labor, early breastfeeding support, and more.

Simonds, W., B. Katz Rothman, and B. M. Norman. 2008. *Laboring On: Birth in Transition in the United States.* London: Routledge.

This book is an updated and expanded version of Rothman's book *In Labor.* In this book, Rothman and colleagues build on her previous works on the subjects of birth and pregnancy and provide a current overview of the changing landscape of birth in the United States. From chapter 1, "Laboring Then: The Political History of Maternity Care in the United States," to chapters on becoming a midwife and practicing midwifery, to considering women as obstetricians and labor and delivery nurses, *Laboring On* is a comprehensive volume that examines the social and political aspects of giving birth from a feminist perspective in the United States.

Stoller Shaw, N. 1974. *Forced Labor.* Oxford, UK, and New York: Pergamon.

This book is a study and analysis of giving birth in the hospital. The author conducted extensive sociological research in various hospital institutions, beginning in 1967, with the goal to understand the process of giving birth in an American hospital and to see how the institution shapes the experience, behavior, and emotions of the patients. This is one of the first books to describe what the medicalization of childbirth looks like in hospitals in the United States.

Summers, A. K. 2014. *Pregnant BUTCH*. Berkeley, CA: Soft Skull Press, an imprint of Counterpoint.
This book is a graphic novel based on the author's own experience of being a self-described pregnant butch lesbian. Using humor and wit, this book explores the experience of navigating pregnancy as a non-gender-conforming person and the intersections between pregnancy, birth, gender, and sexuality.

Susie, D. A. 1988. *In the Way of Our Grandmothers: A Cultural View of Twentieth-Century Midwifery in Florida*. Athens: University of Georgia Press.
This book tells the story of Florida midwifery in the twentieth century, how traditional midwives were subjected to tightened training and licensing restrictions by the state and a burgeoning obstetrics profession that eventually ended with the revoking of their licenses and the attempted eradication of traditional midwifery, only to be eventually replaced by state-sanctioned nurse midwifery. This book tells the stories of the midwives by the people who remember them.

Ulrich, L. T. 1990. *A Midwife's Tale: The Life of Martha Ballard, Based on Her Diary, 1785–1812*. New York: Vintage Books.
The author is a renowned historian who bases the narrative of the book on the diaries of a midwife who lived in a small Maine town. She was the mother to 9 of her own children, and in her career as a midwife, she helped other women birth 816 babies. This book was the winner of the Pulitzer Prize and was made into a film.

Washington, H. A. 2008. *Medical Apartheid: The Dark History of Medical Experimentation on Black Americans from Colonial Times to the Present*. Norwell, MA: Anchor.

> The author recounts the long history of abuses enacted on African Americans by the medical establishment in the United States. The author argues that medicine must acknowledge these abuses to understand African American reluctance toward the medical system and to convince African Americans that despite this history of abuse, there are benefits to selective participation in medicine research studies that benefit community health. The book was the winner of multiple awards.

Wilkie, L. A. 2003. *The Archaeology of Mothering: An African American Midwife's Tale*. New York: Routledge.

> In this book, the author, who is an archeologist, constructs a narrative about an African American midwife from the results of an archeological excavation and interviews conducted. The narrative digs into deeper questions about the meaning of motherhood as revealed by the archeological process.

Worth, J., and T. Coates. 2009. *The Midwife: A Memoir of Birth, Joy, and Hard Times*. New York: Penguin Books.

> This book was the basis for the PBS drama TV series *Call the Midwife*. It is the story of a young midwife who practices in the east end of London in the 1950s.

Articles

American College of Nurse-Midwives, Midwives Alliance of North America; National Association of Certified Professional Midwives. 2012. "Supporting Healthy and Normal Physiologic Childbirth: A Consensus Statement by the American College of Nurse-Midwives, Midwives Alliance of North America, and the National Association of Certified Professional Midwives." *Journal of Midwifery & Women's Health* 57(5): 529–532.

This consensus statement represents the work of a task force composed of representatives from three U.S. midwifery organizations whose members are experts on supporting birthing people's innate capacities to birth. The statement calls for an introduction of policies into hospital settings to support normal physiologic birth; comprehensive examination and dissemination of the evidence and care practices supportive of normal physiologic birth; midwifery care as a key strategy to support normal physiologic birth; increasing the midwife workforce and enhancing regulations and funding strategies to support their practice; competency-based, interdisciplinary education programming for maternity health care clinicians and students on the application of care that promotes normal physiologic birth; and the development of a future research agenda on short- and long-term effects of normal physiologic birth.

Attanasio, L. B., F. Alarid-Escudero, and K. B. Kozhumannil. 2019. "Midwife-Led Care and Obstetrician-Led Care for Low-Risk Pregnancies: A Cost Comparison." *Birth: Issues in Perinatal Care* 47(1): 57–66.

This article uses a decision-analytic model of costs, medical procedures during childbirth, and outcomes of care that show different outcomes between midwife-led care and obstetrician-led care. The authors show that a shift from obstetrician-led care to midwife-led care for low-risk pregnancies would be cost beneficial, and of course beneficial for birthing people and families.

Banerjee, A. 2010. "Reorienting the Ethics of Transnational Surrogacy as a Feminist Pragmatist." *The Pluralist* 5(3): 107–127.

In this article, the author critiques the predominant analysis used to discuss surrogacy and proposes a new feminist, pragmatist theoretical framework to consider surrogacy in the transnational circumstance.

Berkowitz, D. 2008. "A Sociohistorical Analysis of Gay Men's Procreative Consciousness." *Journal of GLBT Family Studies* 3(2–3): 157–190.

>   This is a qualitative study that argues that to understand gay men's perception about becoming fathers and parenthood, it is important to understand the social and historical contexts of the men's lives, which are rapidly changing.

Berkowitz, D., and W. Marsiglio. 2007. "Gay Men: Negotiating Procreative, Father, and Family Identities." *Journal of Marriage and Family* 69(2): 366–381.

>   This qualitative study explores gay male "reproductive consciousness" and argues that men's consciousness evolves over time and is shaped by institutions and emerging structural changes in reproductive technology as well as their own experiences in negotiating with partners, birth mothers, and more.

Black Women Scholars and the Research Working Group of the Black Mamas Matter Alliance. 2020. "Black Maternal Health Research Re-Envisioned: Best Practices for the Conduct of Research With, For, and By Black Mamas." *Harvard Law and Policy Review* 14: 393–415.

>   In this groundbreaking article, the authors provide an overview of a forthcoming report entitled "Black Maternal Health Research Re-Envisioned: Recommendations for Improving Research on Maternity Care for Black Mamas." The report details principles that should underpin the ethical design of clinical, epidemiological, health services, and public health research, specifically, with, for, and by Black Mamas.

Bor, S. E. 2013. "Lucy's Two Babies: Framing the First Televised Depiction of Pregnancy." *Media History* 19(4): 1–15.

>   This article explores the media's portrayal of Lucille Ball's pregnancy on her television show *I Love Lucy* in 1953.

Ball's pregnancy was the first time the subject had been addressed on American television. This research looks at how the media dealt with the emergence of the topic of pregnancy and childbirth on American television.

Clarke, J., and E. Adashi. 2011. "Perinatal Care for Incarcerated Patients: A 25-Year-Old Woman Pregnant in Jail." *Jama-Journal of the American Medical Association* 305(9): 923–929.
Through the case study of Mrs. A, the authors study the experiences and outcomes of perinatal care for incarcerated women in the American prison system.

Conrad, P. 1992. "Medicalization and Social Control." *Annual Review of Sociology* 18: 209–232.
This article considers the relationship between medicalization and social control by analyzing the emergence of medicalization, demedicalization, and lacunae, among others.

Cottom, T. 2019. "I Was Pregnant and in Crisis. All the Doctors and Nurses Saw Was an Incompetent Black Woman." *Time.* https://time.com/5494404/tressie-mcmillan-cottom -thick-pregnancy-competent/.
In this powerful personal essay, sociologist and 2020 MacArthur fellowship award winner shares her experience of being pregnant and birthing while Black in the United States. Her experience painfully illustrates medical racism, particularly the long history of medicine (and other social institutions) ignoring Black pain.

Davies, J., and C. R. Smith. 1998. "Race, Gender, and the American Mother: Political Speech and the Maternity Episodes of *I Love Lucy* and *Murphy Brown.*" *American Studies* 39(2): 33–63.
In this article, the authors analyze the pregnancy episodes of the television shows *I Love Lucy* and *Murphy Brown.*

The authors argue that these media representations can be read as part of the construction of national identity of femininity and whiteness for women in the United States.

Dunne, G. 2000. "Opting into Motherhood: Lesbians Blurring the Boundaries and Transforming the Meaning of Parenthood and Kinship." *Gender & Society* 14(1): 11–35.

This article looks at the experience of lesbian motherhood and makes an argument that lesbians who have children are not opting into the heteronormative family roles by becoming parents. Instead, lesbian families are refashioning family organizational structures and meanings of kinship and negotiating different gender and sexual roles than heteronormative families.

Eichelberger, K. Y., K. Doll, G. E. Ekpo, and M. L. Zerden. 2016. "Black Lives Matter: Claiming a Space for Evidence-Based Outrage in Obstetrics and Gynecology." *American Journal of Public Health* 106(10): 1771–1772.

In this article, researchers use data to show the significant inequities and disparities Black birthing people face in their reproductive lives. They argue for a professional commitment to evidence-based outrage against a broken racist medical system as foundational response to beginning to address Black birth inequities.

Garwood, E. 2016. "Reproducing the Homonormative Family: Neoliberalism, Queer Theory and Same-Sex Reproductive Law." *Journal of International Women's Studies* 17(2): 5–17.

This article looks at the intersections of culture and economics in regard to same-sex reproduction and neoliberalism. Using analysis of the Human Fertilisation and Embryology Act of 2008 (UK), the author argues that policy is often used to reproduce dominant heteronormative social constructions of family and the limiting effect on queer people and families.

Golden, J. 1996. "From Commodity to Gift: Gender, Class, and the Meaning of Breast Milk in the Twentieth Century." *Historian* 59(1): 75–87.

This article tells the history of breast milk and body commodification throughout the United States in the twentieth century. The author examines the way that breast milk and the body became commodified and then sacralized and shows how discourses about class and gender affect the process and meaning of body commodification and the selling of human milk.

Goode, K., and B. Katz Rothman. 2017. "African American Midwifery, a History and a Lament." *American Journal of Economics and Sociology* 76(1): 65–94.

This article centers the importance of African American midwives to U.S. history. The authors not only present the attempted eradication of African American midwives in the twentieth century but also show that African American midwives have always resisted and persisted. African American midwives are imperative to Reproductive Justice for all people, especially Black birthing people.

Harvard Law Department. 2019. "Barbaric Beyond Bans: How the First Step Act's Shackling Provision Fails to Protect Women.'" *Harvard Civil Rights-Civil Liberties Law Review.* https://harvardcrcl.org/barbaric-beyond-bans-the-first-step-acts-shackling-provision-may-not-protect-women/.

This article explains that while the 2018 First Step Act focused on criminal justice reform includes an important ban on the practice of shackling people during childbirth, it is still inefficient in addressing the depths and pervasiveness of this human rights issue. Shackling of pregnant and birthing people is an area of urgent public health concern and further research.

Howell, E. A., N. Egorova, A. Balbierz, J. Zeitlin, and P. L. Hebert. 2016. "Black-White Differences in Severe Maternal Morbidity and Site of Care." *American Journal of Obstetrics and Gynecology* 214(1). https://doi.org/10.1016/j.ajog.2015.08.019.
This article looks at severe maternal morbidity and how hospital locations play a role in the care outcome for Black birthing people. Like maternal mortality, Black people experience maternal morbidity at much higher rates in the United States.

Imogen, T., and L. Baraitser. 2013. "Private View, Public Birth: Making Feminist Sense of the New Visual Culture of Child-birth." *Studies in the Maternal* 5(2): 1–27.
This article considers the last three decades of media representation of pregnancy and childbirth. The authors propose that there has been relatively little new feminist scholarship that relates this new visual culture of childbirth to the earlier feminist discourse of the taboo of the representation of pregnancy. The authors focus their attention on two new sites of representations: birth reality TV and the birthright art collection for their analysis.

Kline, K. 2007. "Midwife Attended Births in Prime-Time Television: Craziness, Controlling Bitches, and Ultimate Capitulation." *Women and Language* 30(1): 20–29.
In this article, the author considers three television depictions of midwife-attended births. The author makes the argument that although, on the surface, the narratives were providing an alternative representation normally presented as highly medicalized birth, the representations actually depicted the midwives and birth in a way that undermined the Midwives Model of Care and reinforced the dominant medicalized version of birth usually seen on televisions.

Kobrin, F. 1966. "The American Midwife Controversy: A Crisis of Professionalization." *Bulletin of the History of Medicine* 40: 350–378.

In this seminal history of American midwifery and obstetrics, the author shows how the rise of the obstetrics field of medicine was not a natural maturation of the field but instead due to the strategic dismantling of the midwifery industry and proponents of a public health approach to maternity care. Kobrin outlines how obstetricians pushed midwives out of the American business of birth and simultaneously benefited from changing public discourse surrounding maternity.

Kuczynski, A. 2008. "Her Body, My Baby." *New York Times*, November 28.

This article is an autobiographical retelling of the author's experience with infertility, undergoing IVF, and hiring a gestational surrogate.

Leavitt, J. W. 1983. "'Science' Enters the Birthing Room: Obstetrics in America since the Eighteenth Century." *Journal of American History* 70(2): 281–304.

In this article, the author collects data from various sources, including medical records, autobiographies, and diaries, to look at how births were affected by the entrance of physicians into the birthing room around the 1760s. The author concludes that for the first 170 years after physicians entered into the birthing room, they did more to harm than help birthing people.

Lu, M. C., M. Kotelchuck, V. Hogan, L. Jones, K. Wright, and N. Halfon. 2010. "Closing the Black-White Gap in Birth Outcomes: A Life-Course Approach." *Ethnicity & Disease* 20: S2-62-76.

In this article, the authors address the disparities between Black and white birth outcomes in the United States. They propose that the public health discourse has unsuccessfully focused on individual risk assessment and access to prenatal care to address these disparities. The authors present a 12-step life course approach to better address the disparities.

Lu, M. C. 2010. "We Can Do Better: Improving Perinatal Health in America." *Journal of Women's Health (2002)* 19(3): 569–574.
In this article, the author argues that the United States—the country that spends the highest amount of money on health care in the world and consistently scores lowest on infant and maternal mortality rates—needs to do better in working to improve perinatal health outcomes. The author concludes that an approach that includes a larger social analysis, such as the life course perspective and the ecological model, would be better suited to improve health outcomes than an approach that solely focuses on individual needs and risk reduction.

Lu, M. C., and C. Halfon. 2003. "Racial and Ethnic Disparities in Birth Outcomes: A Life-Course Perspective." *Maternal and Child Health Journal* 7(1): 13–30.
The authors of this article seek to answer questions about the consistent racial disparities between Black and white levels of infant mortality in the United States. They conduct extensive research through the literature on the subject and develop two longitudinal models to be examined within a life course perspective. The researchers conclude that to better understand the disparities, future research needs to take a nuanced and life course perspective that includes many factors through a woman's life.

Luce, A., M. Cash, V. Hundley, H. Cheyne, E. Van Teijlingen, and C. Angell. 2016. "'Is It Realistic?' The Portrayal of Pregnancy and Childbirth in the Media." *BMC Pregnancy and Childbirth* 16(38): 40–49.
This article is an examination of the representation of childbirth in the television media. The authors ask questions

about the impact of the oftentimes overly dramatic, medicalized, and trauma-laden television births on the understanding of people's expectations of physiologic birth. The authors identify three areas of interest: medicalization of birth, people using media to educate themselves about birth, and lack of representation of physiologic birth in media.

MacDonald, T., J. Noel-Weiss, D. West, M. Walks, M. Biener, A. Kibbe, and E. Myler. 2016. "Transmasculine Individuals' Experiences with Lactation, Chestfeeding, and Gender Identity: A Qualitative Study." *BMC Pregnancy and Childbirth* 16(106): 106.

In this article, the authors interview transmasculine people about their experiences surrounding birth and infant feeding and provide suggestions for health care providers that will help them provide more competent care for transmasculine people.

MacTavish, J. 2011. "Supporting LGBTQ Families: A Brief Cultural Competency Guide for Childbirth Educators and Doulas." *International Journal of Childbirth Education* 26(3): 7–10.

This article gives insight for birth workers to develop LGBTQ cultural competency. The author presents some of the challenges that LGBTQ pregnant people and families may face and provides suggestions for working with LGBTQ families, such as using culturally inclusive language and intentionally using materials that represent LGBTQ people and families.

Manley, M. H., A. E. Goldberg, L. E. Ross, J. C. Gonsiorek, M. E. Brewster, A. L. Brimhall, and A. Pollitt. 2018. "Invisibility and Involvement: LGBTQ Community Connections among Plurisexual Women during Pregnancy and Postpartum." *Psychology of Sexual Orientation and Gender Diversity* 5(2): 169–181.

In this qualitative longitudinal study, researchers ask questions seeking to understand plurisexual (individuals attracted to more than one gender) women's involvement with LGBTQ communities before, during, and after childbirth and seek ways to build community involvement and support.

Markens, S. 2012. "The Global Reproductive Health Market: U.S. Media Framings and Public Discourses about Transnational Surrogacy." *Social Science & Medicine* 74(11): 1745–1753.

This article is the first empirical study on how the U.S. media covers surrogacy. The author's analysis considers the exploitation versus opportunity discourses surrounding surrogacy. The author concludes that nationalized, racialized, and classed embodiments experience a hierarchy of reproductive values depending on location and argues that an intersectional analysis of assisted reproductive technology and surrogacy is important for a complex understanding of the discourses.

Markens, S. 2017. "'I'm Not Sure if They Speak to Everyone about This Option': Analyzing Disparate Access to and Use of Genetic Health Services in the US from the Perspective of Genetic Counselors." *Critical Public Health* 27(1): 111–124.

In this article, the authors look at the factors that inhibit certain populations from using genetic medical technologies and suggest that these factors, whether patient centered or structural, could contribute to larger health disparities in the U.S. population.

Martin, L. J. 2010. "Anticipating Infertility: Egg Freezing, Genetic Preservation, and Risk." *Gender & Society* 24(4): 526–545.

This article focuses on "anticipated infertility" and the use of reproductive technologies. People who are not infertile may take anticipatory steps to deal with possible future infertility. The author looks at how this anticipatory infertility interacts with the discourses surrounding medicalization.

Martin, L. J. 2009. "Reproductive Tourism in the Age of Globalization." *Globalizations* 6(2): 249–263.

The author looks at the intersections of reproductive tourism—the practice of going abroad to engage in assisted reproductive technologies- and national regulation, consumer desire, and the global market.

Martin, N., and R. Montagne. 2019. "Nothing Protects Black Women from Dying in Pregnancy and Childbirth." *ProPublica*. https://www.propublica.org/article/nothing-protects-black-women-from-dying-in-pregnancy-and-childbirth.

This article is part of ProPublica's Lost Mothers series. This article tells Shalon Irving's story. Shalon Irving was a Black mother who died three weeks after giving birth despite having a dual PhD, high income, and a lieutenant commander ranking in the Commissioned Corps of the U.S. Public Health Service and being an epidemiologist at the Centers for Disease Control and Prevention.

Mongeau, B., H. Smith, and A. Maney. 1961. "The 'Granny' Midwife: Changing Roles and Functions of a Folk Practitioner." *American Journal of Sociology* 66(5): 497–505.

This article documents the historical changes in African American midwifery in the southern United States.

Morris, T., and K. McInerney. 2010. "Media Representations of Pregnancy and Childbirth: An Analysis of Reality Television Programs in the United States." *Birth* 37(2): 134–140.

This analysis of television portrayals of pregnancy and birth suggests that the programs do not give a realistic evidence-based portrayal of birth; instead, they support a narrative that women's bodies are incapable of normal physiologic birth and are in need of medical intervention.

Nordqvist, P. 2015. "'I've Redeemed Myself by Being a 1950s "Housewife"': Parent–Grandparent Relationships in the Context of Lesbian Childbirth." *Journal of Family Issues* 36(4): 480–500. https://doi.org/10.1177/0192513X14563798.

Lesbian families using donor sperm to achieve pregnancy are reshaping heteronormative constructs about family and kinship. This study looks at how grandparents (parents of lesbian mothers) negotiate those kinship changes.

Ocen, P. A. 2012. "Punishing Pregnancy: Race, Incarceration, and the Shackling of Pregnant Prisoners." *California Law Review* 100(5): 1239–1311.

This article argues that to understand the practice and to dissuade the use of shackling of incarcerated pregnant people, it is first necessary to understand the social construction of race and gender that perpetuates this inhuman practice.

Petrovska, K., A. Sheehan, and C. S. E. Homer. 2017. "Media Representations of Breech Birth: A Prospective Analysis of Web-Based News Reports." *Journal of Midwifery & Women's Health* 62(4): 434–441.

This is the first research to look into the media's representation of breech childbirth (when the fetus is positioned to present the feet first) and the effect on people's perception of breech birth.

Roberts, D. E. 2009. "Race, Gender, and Genetic Technologies: A New Reproductive Dystopia?" *Signs* 34(4): 783–804. https://doi.org/10.1086/597132.

Building on earlier feminist discourses about reproductive dystopias involving genetic technologies and stratified reproductive hierarchies privileging white women, the author argues for a new reproductive dystopia discourse that critically examines the intersections of the reproductive technologies, neoliberalism, and racism.

Roeder, A. 2019. "America Is Failing Its Black Mothers." *Harvard Public Health*. https://www.hsph.harvard.edu/magazine/magazine_article/america-is-failing-its-black-mothers/.
This article discusses the high maternal mortality in the United States and the racial inequities that endanger Black women regardless of economic or educational status.

Rothman, B. Katz. 1978. "Childbirth as Negotiated Reality." *Symbolic Interaction* 1(2): 124–137.
This article looks at birth as a socially constructed and defined event that is controlled by a medical perspective. It also looks at the role of childbirth education in reproducing the normative medical perspective on birth and considers an alternative nonmedical birthing construction.

Ryan, M. 2013. "The Gender of Pregnancy: Masculine Lesbians Talk about Reproduction." *Journal of Lesbian Studies* 17(2): 119–133.
This article examines how heterosexism and patriarchy have created social ideologies for all women. Expectations include that all women will become pregnant and that pregnancy is a femininely embodied event. It then investigates how these expectations create complexities for masculine-embodied lesbians in their perception of their own possible future pregnancies.

Smith, W. E. 1951. "Nurse Midwife Maude Callen Eases Pain of Birth and Death." LIFE, December 3.
This classic photo essay features nurse-midwife Maude Callen as she provided midwifery care. Maude Callen was a revered grand midwife.

Suter, V., E. Nethery, M. L. Kopas, H. Wurz, K. Sitcov, and A. B. Caughey. 2019. "Comparison of Midwifery and Obstetric Care in Low-Risk Hospital Births." *Obstetrics and Gynecology* 134(5): 1056–1065.

This article compares midwife and obstetrician labor practices and birth outcomes in people who have low-risk pregnancies that are delivered in the hospital. Researchers found that greater intervention of midwifery care may reduce labor intervention in low-risk pregnancies.

Takeshita, C. 2017. "Countering Technocracy: 'Natural' Birth in *The Business of Being Born* and *Call the Midwife*." *Feminist Media Studies* 17(3): 332–346.

In this article, the author argues that while most media representations of childbirth reproduce a medicalized normative model, these two media representations produce nonmedicalized media images and promote a normalized view of midwifery care and a critique of the medically dominated childbirth.

Thomas, M.-P., G. Ammann, E. Brazier, P. Noyes, and A. May-bank. 2017. "Doula Services within a Healthy Start Program: Increasing Access for an Underserved Population." *Maternal and Child Health Journal* 21(Suppl 1): 59–64.

This article looks at the effects of doula care on maternal mortality, morbidity, and poor birth outcomes. This article assesses the impacts of New York City's Department of Health and Mental Hygiene Department's introduction of the By My Side Birth Support Program, which provided doula care to pregnant, birthing, and postpartum women.

Tunc, T. E. 2010. "The Mistress, the Midwife, and the Medical Doctor: Pregnancy and Childbirth on the Plantations of the Antebellum American South, 1800–1860." *Women's History Review* 19(3): 395–419.

This article examines the complex relationships between plantation mistresses, enslaved midwives, and medical doctors during the antebellum period. In particular, it examines the effects of pregnancy and birth on these complex social relationships.

Vedam, S., K. Stoll, T. K. Taiwo, N. Rubashkin, M. Cheyney, N. Strauss, M. McLemore, et al. 2019. "The Giving Voice to Mothers Study: Inequity and Mistreatment during Pregnancy and Childbirth in the United States." *Reproductive Health* 16(77). https://doi.org/10.1186/s12978-019-0729-2.

This article used an online cross-sectional survey to capture the lived experiences of maternity care in diverse populations. The authors found that people of color are more likely to experience mistreatment when birth occurs in hospitals and among those with social, economic, and health challenges.

Vedam, S., K. Stoll, M. MacDorman, E. Declercq, R. Cramer, M. Cheyney, T. Fisher, et al. 2018. "Mapping Integration of Midwives across the United States: Impact on Access, Equity, and Outcomes." *PLoS ONE* 13(2): e0192523. https://doi.org /10.1371/journal.pone.0192523.

This study looks at the integration and impacts of midwives across the United States. Wherever there are midwives, there is better care for birthing people.

Vedam, S., K. Stoll, N. Rubashkin, K. Martin, Z. Miller-Vedam, H. Hayes-Klein, G. Jolicoeur, et al. 2017. "The Mothers on Respect (MOR) Index: Measuring Quality, Safety, and Human Rights in Childbirth." *SSM—Population Health* 3(C): 201–210.

The Mothers on Respect Index is a tool used to measure birthing people's perception of comfort, respect, racism, and discrimination when interacting in the patient-provider relationship during pregnancy and birth care. The authors believe that the introduction of the MOR Index to institutions could have positive impacts on birthing people's experience of respectful care.

Wakeel F., W. P. Witt, L. E. Wisk, M. C. Lu, and S. M. Chao. 2014. "Racial and Ethnic Disparities in Personal Capital during Pregnancy: Findings from the 2007 Los Angeles Mommy and Baby (LAMB) Study." *Maternal Child Health Journal* 18: 209–222.
    This article explores the role that personal capital, defined as "protective resources that a woman may draw upon during pregnancy," has on the effects of maternal and infant outcomes.

Wilton, T. 1999. "Towards an Understanding of the Cultural Roots of Homophobia in Order to Provide a Better Midwifery Service for Lesbian Clients." *Midwifery* 15(3): 154–164.
    This analysis of homophobia in midwifery culture identifies themes that may be used to understand and deconstruct homophobia to provide lesbian clients with better midwifery care.

Reports

Amnesty International. 2010. *Deadly Delivery: The Maternal Healthcare Crisis in the USA*. London: Amnesty International. https://www.amnestyusa.org/files/pdfs/deadlydelivery.pdf.
    This report is based on research conducted by Amnesty International to analyze the maternal health care system in the United States from a human rights perspective and give suggestions for improvement. They interviewed hundreds of women about their birthing experiences and federal workers working in the Division of Health and Human Services and reviewed media reports of maternal and infant deaths.

Avery, M., A. Bell., D. Bingham, M. Corry, S. Delbanco, S. Leavitt Gullo, H. Catherine, et al. 2018. *Blueprint for Advancing High Value Maternity Care through Physiologic Childbearing*. Washington, DC: National Partnership for Women and Families.
    This report is a collaborative work designed as a guide to strategies developed to increase high-value maternity

care systems to improve healthy maternal and infant outcomes. The approach is to provide appropriate care for low-risk healthy women during pregnancy who are often provided more specialized care than necessary in the maternal health care system and may as a result be experiencing preventable harm from the system.

Bey, A., A. Brill, C. Porchia-Albert, M. Gradilla, and N. Strauss. *Advancing Birth Justice: Community-Based Doula Models as a Standard of Care for Ending Racial Disparities.* n.p.: Ancient Song Doula Services, Village Birth International, and Every Birth Matters. Accessed March 25, 2019. https://everymothercounts .org/wp-content/uploads/2019/03/Advancing-Birth-Justice -CBD-Models-as-Std-of-Care-3-25-19.pdf.

In 2018, the State of New York introduced a Medicaid doula pilot program in an effort to address racial inequities in childbirth and end maternal mortality in the state. This report defines a difference between "traditional" pay-for-services doula care and community-based doula care that is usually no or low fee. The report looks at New York's pilot doula program and suggests successful ways a community-based doula model can be advanced to support the goals of the policy and provide wider access to doula care for low-income communities and communities of color.

Black Mamas Matter Alliance and Center for Reproductive Rights. 2016. *Black Mamas Matter: Advancing the Human Right to Safe and Respectful Maternal Health Care.* New York: Center for Reproductive Rights. https://Blackmamasmatter.org /resources/toolkits/.

This report is a toolkit created by a collaboration of the authoring organizations. The toolkit provides advocacy tools and resources for state health care officials and policy makers. The purpose of the toolkit is to enable policy makers to work toward a human rights–based approach to improving maternal health care for Black people in the United States. This toolkit is a classic text in the canon of Reproductive Justice literature.

Cole, H. E., P. X. Rojas, and J. Joseph. *National Perinatal Taskforce Report: Building a Movement to Birth a More Just and Loving World.* Accessed March 2018. https://perinataltaskforce .com/heads-up-maternal-justice-npt-2018-report-out-now/.
The National Perinatal Task Force is a grassroots organization founded by midwife Jennie Joseph and other health activists. This report addresses the crisis in maternal and infant health in the United States, especially for Black people. The report identifies areas of need, introduces a system of "perinatal safe spots," and offers solutions and suggestions for all health care providers.

Finkelstein, A., S. M. Dougall, A. Kintominas, and A. Olsen. *Surrogacy Law and Policy in the United States: A National Conversation Informed by Global Lawmaking.* Accessed November 12, 2020. https://web.law.columbia.edu/sites/default/files/microsites /gender-sexuality/files/columbia_sexuality_and_gender_law_clinic _-_surrogacy_law_and_policy_report_-_june_2016.pdf.
This report reviews the laws and regulations of international and U.S. surrogacy. It then considers the issues surrounding the legalization of surrogacy.

Hill, I., L. Dubay, B. Courtot, S. Benatar, B. Garrett, F. Blavin, E. Howell, et al. 2018. *Strong Start for Mothers and Newborns Evaluation: Year 5 Project Synthesis.* Washington, DC: Urban Institute. https://downloads.cms.gov/files/cmmi/strongstart -prenatal-finalevalrpt-v1.pdf.
This report evaluates findings from the survey of the Strong Starts for Mothers and Newborn Initiative. The initiative aimed to improve health care outcomes for mothers and infants who received Medicaid and participated in

the children's health insurance program. This is the final report of the program.

National Academies of Sciences, Engineering, and Medicine; Health and Medicine Division; Division of Behavioral and Social Sciences and Education; Board on Children, Youth, and Families; Committee on Assessing Health Outcomes by Birth Settings. 2020. *Birth Settings in America: Outcomes, Quality, Access, and Choice.* Edited by E. P. Backes and S. C. Scrimshaw. Washington, DC: National Academies Press.

> This report identifies ways to improve childbirth services in all birth settings. It determines that childbearing people having informed choice regarding birth settings and the removal of barriers to community birth are essential to improving birth outcomes and experiences, along with greater coordination and integration of maternity care providers in the system.

Sakala, C., E. R. Declercq, J. M. Turon, and M. P. Corry. 2018. *Listening to Mothers in California: A Population-Based Survey of Women's Childbearing Experiences, Full Survey Report.* Washington, DC: National Partnership for Women & Families.

> This report is the result of a large survey of California childbearing women. The purpose of the survey was to gather information about the women's perception of their prenatal, pregnancy, birth, and postpartum experiences to provide information to those who are interested in improving maternal and infant health care. The survey focused on women who gave birth in hospitals.

Internet Resources and Mixed Media

American Civil Liberties Union. 2012. "State Standards for Pregnancy-Related Health Care and Abortion for Women in Prison—Map." Last modified July 2012. https://www.aclu.org

/state-standards-pregnancy-related-health-care-and-abortion
-women-prison-0.
    This website hosts an interactive map that provides access
    to research that looks at state, national, and federal poli-
    cies that specifically deal with pregnant prisoners as posted
    on department corrections websites and databases.

Ancient Song Doula Services. n.d. "Reclaiming the Ancient
Principles of Birthing." Accessed January 29, 2019. https://
www.ancientsongdoulaservices.com/.
    Ancient Song offers quality doula care to women of
    color and low-income women in New York City. Ancient
    Song engages in Reproductive Justice and policy and
    advocacy work to improve the health outcomes and ineq-
    uities faced by birthing people in marginalized commu-
    nities.

Ankush. 2018. "Chestfeeding." Gender Confirmation Center
(blog). https://www.genderconfirmation.com/blog/chestfeeding/.
    This webpage offers valuable information and education
    about chestfeeding.

Asher, W., dir. 1953. "Lucy Goes to the Hospital." I Love Lucy,
Episode 16. Written by Jess Oppenheimer, Madelyn Pugh,
and Bob Carrol Jr. Featuring Lucille Ball, Desi Arnaz, Vivian
Vance, and William Frawley. Aired on January 19, 1953, on
CBS.
    This episode of I Love Lucy was the first time that preg-
    nancy and birth had been depicted on network American
    television.

Balmès, T., dir. 2010. Babies. StudioCanal. DVD.
    This French documentary film by Thomas Balmès follows
    four birthing people from very different cultures through
    their first year after birth.

Being Serena. 2018. Season 1, episodes 1–5. Produced by M. Shapiro, M. Antinoro, and W. Staeger. Home Box Office, Inc.
This documentary about the life of superstar tennis player Serena Williams covers her experiences of pregnancy and birth, including her near-death experience in the hospital after giving birth and being neglected by her physicians.

Birth for Every Body. n.d. "About Gender." Accessed January 28, 2019. http://www.birthforeverybody.org/what-we-do/.
This webpage is a list of LGBTQ resources that explore the intersections of gender, pregnancy, and birth. The page is a learning resources for providers, parents, and allies of LGBTQ, transgender, and gender non-conforming people.

The Birth Place Lab. n.d. "Tools." Accessed January 28, 2019. https://www.birthplacelab.org/tools/.
This website provides access to tools of measurement to improve perinatal health care. The tools include The Birth Place Research Quality Index (ResQu Index), Mother's Autonomy in Decision Making (MADM) scale, and the Mothers on Respect (MOR) Index.

Buonaugurio, S., dir. 2008. *Pregnant in America.* Bella Media Productions. DVD.
This documentary is about the birth of the filmmaker's daughter. The filmmaker and his wife wanted to make a documentary that looked into the medicalization of American perinatal health care and to document their choice to have a planned home birth.

Centers for Disease Control and Prevention (CDC). 2019. "Data and Statistics." https://www.cdc.gov/reproductivehealth/data_stats/index.htm.
This webpage provides access to data and statistics collected by the Centers for Disease Control and Prevention's

surveillance systems concerning infant and maternal health and mortality.

Chocolate Milk. 2019. http://www.chocolatemilkdoc.com/.
Chocolate Milk: The Documentary is an exploration of over 40 years of racial disparity in breastfeeding rates among white and Black women in the United States. Black Breastfeeding Week (see Chapter 7) was started to raise awareness about this issue. Increased breastfeeding among Black women could have a significant impact on decreasing infant mortality and preventing disease-related diseases. However, these are systemic issues, such as a lactation field that is not racially/ethnically representative, food deserts in many Black communities, and a lack of media portrayals normalizing and celebrating breastfeeding in general, much less among Black women. Told through the narratives of three Black women—a new mother, a midwife, and a WIC lactation educator—the film seeks to answer the long-standing question of why more Black women are not breastfeeding.

Davenport, N., dir. 2013. *First Comes Love*. Home Box Office, Inc. DVD.
Filmmaker Nina Davenport chronicles her path to becoming a single parent by choice.

The Doula Project. 2019. "About Us." https://www.doulaproject .net/.
The Doula Project is a nonprofit organization in New York City that offers support for people across the spectrum of pregnancy.

Elson, V., dir. 2009. *Laboring under an Illusion: Mass Media Childbirth vs. the Real Thing*. CreateSpace. DVD.
In this film, anthropologist Vicki Elson contrasts 100 fictional and real depictions of birth as a way of exploring the question of how media depictions of birth influence our ideas about pregnancy and birth.

Epstein, A., dir. 2008. *Business of Being Born*. Barranca Productions. DVD.

This documentary film explores how business, technology, and the medicalization of birth has affected birth in the United States and explores producer Ricki Lake's experience of home birth.

Epstein, A., dir. 2012. *More Business of Being Born*. Alchemy. DVD.

Part 2 of the documentary *Business of Being Born* continues the conversation about childbirth and discusses participants' home birth experiences.

Ewing, H., and R. Grady, dirs. 2010. *12th and Delaware*. Home Box Office, Inc. DVD.

This television movie documents the corner of 12th and Delaware in Fort Pierce, Florida, where an abortion clinic and a Catholic pregnancy center are located on the same corner. It won a Peabody Award that same year "for its poignant portrait of women facing exceedingly difficult decisions at a literal intersection of opposing ideologies."

Family Equity Council. n.d. Accessed January 29, 2019. https://www.familyequality.org/.

The Family Equity Council works through advocacy, education, and community building to increase legal and lived equity for LGBTQ families. Their work centers love, justice, family and equality.

Henze, C., dir. 2014. *40 Weeks*. GathrFilms. DVD.

This documentary captures the weekly experiences of pregnant people. Their diverse experiences, approaches, and challenges will educate the audience through common pregnancy milestones, including finding out they are pregnant, increasing hormone levels, sonograms and the first heartbeat, going public, miscarriage risks, amniocentesis and genetic reviews, premature birth survival, completed lung development, and finally preparation for the birth.

Hodon, S. 2017. "Measuring Women's Autonomy and Respect during Maternity Care." *Maternal Health Task Force* (blog). May 28, 2017. https://www.mhtf.org/2017/05/18/measuring -womens-autonomy-and-respect-during-maternity-care/.
This blog post introduces the Mothers on Respect (MOR) Index and the Mother's Autonomy in Decision Making (MADM) scale. These two measurement tools were developed to measure the quality of women's experiences during maternity care.

Human Rights Campaign. n.d. "Explore Parenting." Accessed January 28, 2019. https://www.hrc.org/resources/parenting.
This webpage hosted by the Human Rights Campaign is a resource list for LGBTQ parents-to-be, including information on ways to become parents as well as tools for LGBTQ issues.

In The Womb. Season 1, Episodes 1–8. Created by Toby Macdonald. National Geographic Partners. Aired March 6, 2005.
Advanced technology provides ultrasound images of the developmental phases of a fetus.

Jacobs, R., dir. 2008. *A Sentence for Two*. Angels Flight Productions. DVD.
This documentary follows three women in an Oregon prison who are facing birth and separation from their babies. It also looks at the prison nursery alternative that some prisons are starting to open as the numbers of women in prison keep rising.

Jordan, G., dir. 2001. *Midwives*. Columbia Tristar Television. TV Movie.
This Lifetime movie stars Sissy Spacek and is based on Chris Bohjalian's novel *Midwives*.

Kelly, R. 2018. "How the MOMMA Act Will Help to Reverse America's Rising Maternal Mortality Rate." Media Center, June 5. https://robinkelly.house.gov/media-center/in-the-news/how-the-momma-act-will-help-to-reverse-america-s-rising-maternal-mortality.

This webpage from Congresswoman Robin Kelly's website presents the MOMMA Act, a piece of legislature introduced by Congresswoman Kelly to address the maternal mortality crisis in the United States.

Kelton, J., and R. Hopkins. n.d. *If These Ovaries Could Talk.* Podcast, MP3 audio. Accessed January 12, 2019. https://www.ovariestalk.com/.

This podcast is hosted by two lesbians who talk about navigating issues of pregnancy, childbirth, parenting, and more as queer families in a heteronormative world.

Kirschenbaum, S., dir. 2018. *These Are My Hours.* Swell Dudela Films. DVD.

This film features Emily Graham's physical, emotional, and psychological experiences while giving birth.

La Leche League. n.d. "Transgender & Non-Binary Parents." Breastfeeding Info. Accessed January 28, 2019. https://www.llli.org/breastfeeding-info/transgender-non-binary-parents/.

This webpage offers educational support resources for transgender and non-binary parents about lactation and chestfeeding.

Lamm, S., and M. Wigmore, dirs. 2013. *Birth Story: Ina May Gaskin & the Farm Midwives.* Ghost Robot.

This documentary is about Ina May Gaskin and her fellow midwives who lived in a commune in the 1970s and learned how to catch babies.

MacDonald, T. 2018. "Transgender Parenting and Chest/ Breastfeeding." KellyMom. https://kellymom.com/bf/got-milk /transgender-parents-chestbreastfeeding/.
> This webpage post is authored by transgender health researcher Trevor MacDonald, who became the first transmasculine person to be accredited as an La Leche League leader. This article discusses chestfeeding for transmasculine parents and their care persons.

National Birth Equity Collaborative. n.d. Accessed January 21, 2021. http://birthequity.org/.
> National Birth Equity Collaborative is an organization that works to reduce Black maternal and infant mortality in the United States by engaging in research, advocacy, and family-centered collaborations.

Queer Birth Project. n.d. Home page. Accessed January 29, 2019. https://www.queerbirthproject.org/.
> The Queer Birth Project is an organization the provides education and support for queer families and their birth professionals during pregnancy, childbirth, and early parenting.

Richardson, A., dir. 2011. *Babies behind Bars*. Discovery, Inc.
> This documentary looks into the experiences of women who give birth in prison and the development of prison nurseries. The Indiana Women's Prison is one of the prisons that allows women who give birth to keep their babies while serving their sentences.

Romper's Doula Diaries. 2019. "Doula Diaries." Facebook. https://www.facebook.com/RompersDoulaDiaries/.
> Romper media has created a web series about doulas and people giving birth.

Shannon, L., dir. 2017. *Death by Delivery: The Naked Truth.* Aired on March 8, 2017, on Fusion TV.

This film documents the systemic racism in the American perinatal health care system and the calamitous effects on Black women.

SisterSong. n.d. "SisterSong." Accessed January 29, 2019. https://www.sistersong.net/mission/.

Created in 1997, SisterSong Women of Color Reproductive Justice Collective is a Southern–based national organization that works to improve systems and institutional policies that affect the reproductive rights of women of color.

Stony, G., dir. 1953. *All My Babies . . . a Midwife's Own Story.* Center for Mass Communication of Columbia University Press.

This film tells the story of Miss Mary Coley, an African American midwife in rural Georgia who started her career more than a half century ago. Made as a demonstration film for illiterate "granny" midwives, the film's production was sponsored by the Georgia Department of Public Health and provided the noted filmmaker access to the lives and work of the midwives. The film became a standard part of medical school curriculum because of its safe depiction of birth and was widely distributed by the World Health Organization and UNESCO.

Zoila Pérez, M. 2017. "How Racism Harms Pregnant Women— And What Can Help." TED Talk, March 8. YouTube video, 12:25. https://youtu.be/ktOeFgmdIAo.

Miriam Zoila Perez is a doula turned journalist who explores the relationship between race, class, and illness and tells of a radically compassionate prenatal care program that can help with the stress pregnant people of color experience every day.

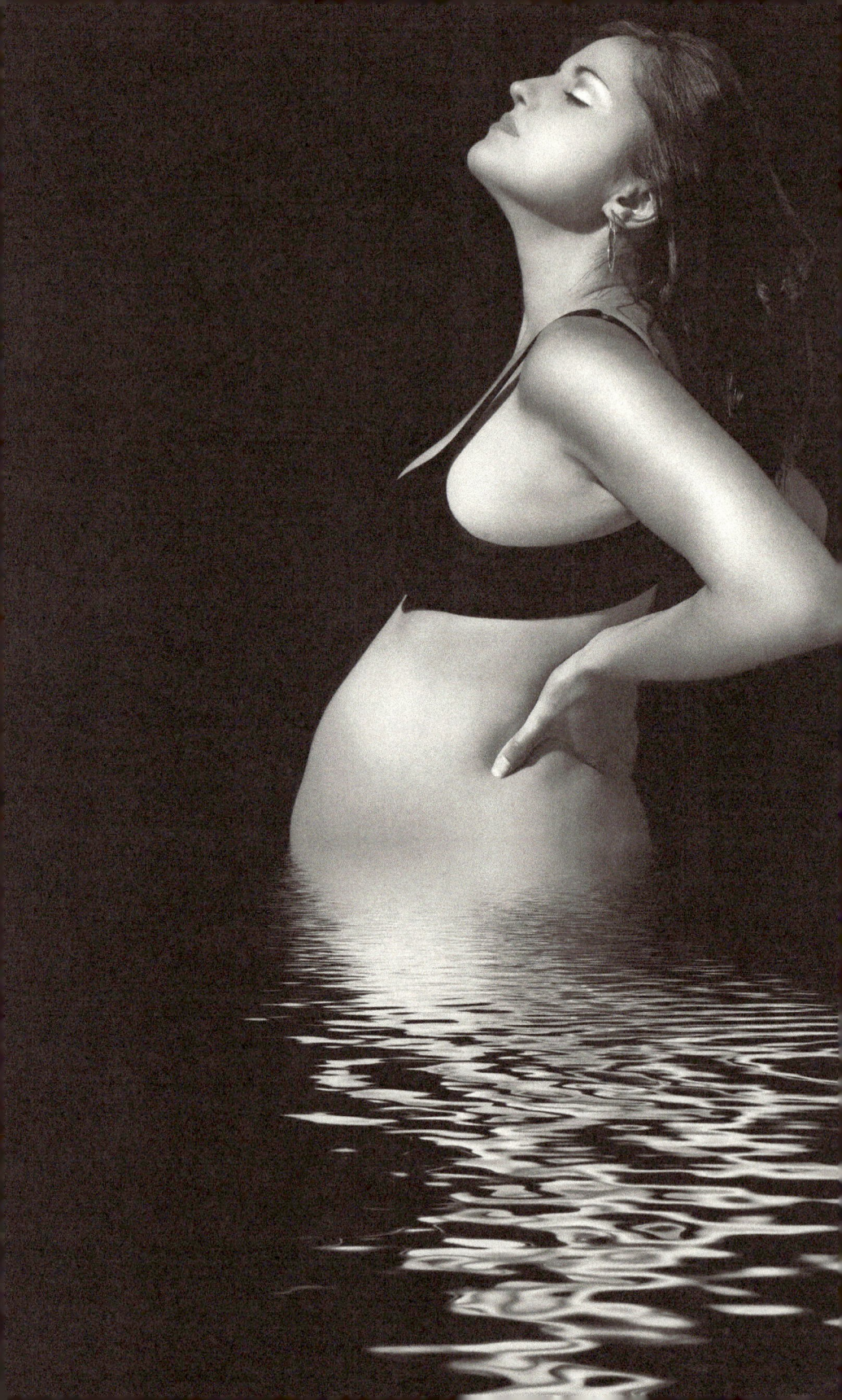

Introduction

Given humans' upright stance and relatively large heads, we are among the very few mammals who do not give birth alone. Every human community has seen the development of a skilled practitioner in birth assistance, known in English as *midwife*, from the Old English word for "with woman." This book focuses on the American experience of pregnancy and birth. Indigenous people had midwives. Black people had a rich history of midwifery on the African continent before being enslaved; they brought midwifery with them. But early on in the history of the United States, medicine as a profession took root and began encroaching on the field of midwifery. Over time, pregnancy and childbirth have become increasingly medicalized, and at this point in time, there is both cooperation and competition between midwives, physicians, and birth workers others over the management and control of pregnancy and birth. This chapter summarizes some of the important events that have occurred in the history of pregnancy and childbirth in the United States.

1847 The American Medical Association (AMA) is founded as a result of a report written by Dr. Nathan Smith Davis calling for a national medical convention. At the time, Davis was the chairman of the Committee on Correspondence relative to medical education and examination. The AMA was the first organization

A pregnant person standing in water. (Marilyn Barbone/Dreamstime.com)

of its kind in the world. It was formed as a national professional medical organization with goals of scientific advancement, new standards for medical education, medical ethics, and improved public health. This organization established the first national code for medical practice, the AMA Code of Medical Ethics, and educated individuals on the dangers of patented medicines and worked to regulate their production.

1910 Abraham Flexner publishes an evaluative report on medical education in the United States. Among other things, this report led to the closing of many historically Black medical colleges, the effects of which are still evident with a predominantly white physician workforce today.

1912 The Maternal and Child Health Bureau of Health Resources and Services Administration of the U.S. government is established under President Taft as the federal commitment to addressing maternal and child health. Its mission was to investigate and report on matters pertaining to the welfare of all children among all classes of people.

1916 Planned Parenthood is founded on the revolutionary idea that people should have the proper information and care necessary to live strong, healthy lives and have the families why and how they desire. Margaret Sanger, along with her sister Ethel Byrne and fellow activist Fania Mindell, opened the United States' first birth control clinic in Brownsville, Brooklyn.

1918 Childbirth Connection, formerly known as the Maternity Center Association, is founded as a nonprofit organization that works to improve the overall quality of maternity care. The organization grew out of the Women's City Club of New York City, which consisted of over 2,000 influential women who worked to reduce infant and maternal mortality rates. Through research, education, advocacy, and policy, Childbirth Connection promotes maternity care that is safe and effective and gives a voice to all childbearing women and families.

1921 The Sheppard-Towner Act, also known as the Promotion of the Welfare and Hygiene of Maternity and Infancy Act, is passed by the U.S. Congress to provide federal funding for maternity and childcare. It was sponsored by both Senator Morris Sheppard of Texas and Representative Horace Mann Towner of Iowa and signed by President Warren G. Harding. This was the first major legislation to exist after the passage of the Nineteenth Amendment, and it played a huge role in the medicalization of pregnancy and birth and regulation of midwifery.

1938 The March of Dimes is founded by President Franklin D. Roosevelt. It was originally known as the National Foundation for Infantile Paralysis, which was created to end polio. Once polio was eradicated, the focus shifted to preventing congenital disabilities and infant mortality.

1949 Virginia Apgar becomes the first woman to hold a full-time professor position at Columbia University College of Physicians and Surgeons, where she starts the first anesthesia division. In 1953, she introduced the Apgar test, the first test that could assess the health of newborn babies. She later worked for the March of Dimes Foundation as the vice president for medical affairs and directed research programs on how to prevent and treat congenital disabilities. Apgar was also one of the first people to bring attention to the issue of premature birth, which is now a main focus of the March of Dimes. Throughout her lifetime, she advocated for universal vaccination for rubella, promoted the effective use of Rh testing to identify causes of hydrops and miscarriage, and became the first woman to hold a faculty position in teratology, the study of congenital disabilities, at the Cornell University School of Medicine. She published over sixty scientific articles and other essays before her death in 1974.

1950 Lamaze is introduced throughout the 1950s by Fernand Lamaze as a method of childbirth involving psychological and physical preparation for pregnant and birthing to help suppress pain and facilitate child delivery without the use of drugs. It involves educating people on the stages of labor and delivery and taught methods for relaxing muscles during labor to lessen pain-increasing tension and anxiety around childbirth.

1951 The American College of Obstetricians and Gynecologists is founded as a professional association of physicians in the United States who specialize in obstetrics and gynecology.

1953 The film *All My Babies: A Midwife's Own Story* is released by George C. Stoney with the purpose of educating U.S. midwives in the South and promoting better cooperation between midwifery and modern health care. The film follows an African American midwife from Albany, Georgia, named Mary Francis Hill Coley, who throughout the mid-twentieth century helped deliver over 3,000 babies.

1955 The American College of Nurse-Midwives is formed in 1955 as the professional organization for certified nurse-midwives and certified midwives.

1955 The Friedman curve is developed by Dr. Friedman, of Columbia University, from a study he had undertaken of 500 first-time people who gave birth at full term. Their labors were plotted on a graph, and the average time it took for a person in the hospital, under the particular and unique circumstances of American hospitalization at that time, to dilate each centimeter was calculated. It has been used as the standard test for rates of cervical dilation and fetal descent during active labor for the past 60 years.

1956 The La Leche League is founded in Franklin Park, Illinois, by a group of seven mothers who wanted to provide help and support with breastfeeding to any interested person. This eventually led to changes in infant care practices, such as promoting partners in the delivery room, returning to home birth for those who want it, and holding newborn babies immediately after birth. The La Leche League has since reached international status and has continued its primary focus of personal sharing of information and encouragement of new parents breastfeeding their babies.

1970   The first publication and founding of *Our Bodies, Ourselves* is created by a group of twelve women from Emmanuel College who met in a workshop called Women and Their Bodies. Their discussions were so fulfilling that they formed a group to research and discuss all they were learning about their bodies and health. They later published a 193-page course booklet entitled *Women and Their Bodies*, later changed to *Our Bodies, Ourselves*.

1971   The American Midwifery Certification Board, formerly the ACNM Certification Council, Inc., is founded as the national certifying body for certified nurse-midwives and certified midwives.

1973   *Roe v. Wade* is a landmark decision by the U.S. Supreme Court in which the court ruled that the due process clause of the Fourteenth Amendment to the U.S. Constitution provides a fundamental "right to privacy" that protects a pregnant person's liberty to choose whether or not to have an abortion.

1978   The first in vitro fertilization baby, or IVF, a medical procedure in which a woman's egg is fertilized by sperm outside of the body, is born on July 15, in Oldham, England. Louise Joy Brown is best known as being the world's first "test-tube baby." Her birth by cesarean section made headlines around the world.

1978   Suzy Myers and a team of passionate activists found the Seattle Midwifery School, which offered the oldest direct-entry midwifery training program. Their mission was to train women's health care providers and provide all people and families with access to care, education, and options to contribute to a happy, healthy, and safe pregnancy, including during birth and the postpartum period.

1982   The Midwives Alliance of North America (MANA) is established as a professional organization for all midwives of all credentials. It grew out of a grassroots coalition of diverse types of midwives from across North America. MANA was created with the desire to establish a professional home for all midwives that would recognize and honor the diversity of educational backgrounds and practice styles within the profession.

1982   The Accreditation Commission for Midwifery Education is officially recognized by the U.S. Department of Education, under health care, as an accrediting agency for nurse-midwifery education.

1983   The American Association of Birth Centers (AABC), formerly known as the Cooperative Birth Center Network, is founded by Childbirth Connection, formerly known as the Maternity Center Association. The AABC promotes and supports birth centers as a means to uphold the rights of healthy people and their families within all communities to birth their children in safe, sensitive, and cost-effective environments with minimal intervention.

1984   The Black Women's Health Imperative (BWHI) is founded as the only national organization solely dedicated to improving the health and wellness of the nation's 21 million Black women and girls, physically, emotionally, and financially. It was founded by Byllye Avery, who was involved in reproductive health care work and wanted to provide an environment in which women could feel comfortable and take control of their own health and well-being. The mission of BWHI is to solve the most pressing issues that affect Black women and girls in the United States through investments in evidence-based strategies to deliver bold new programs and advocate for policies that promote health.

1986   The Baby M custody case becomes the first American court ruling on the validity of surrogacy. Baby M, born March 27, 1986, was the product of a surrogacy agreement between William Stern and Mary Beth Whitehead, whom William and his wife, Elizabeth Stern, found through a newspaper ad. Whitehead was to be inseminated with William's sperm, bring the pregnancy to full term, and then relinquish parental rights to the Sterns. Whitehead relinquished her rights at the birth, but days later, she refused to relinquish her parenthood. The New Jersey court ruled the surrogacy contract invalid but awarded Stern with custody of the child, allowing Whitehead visitation rights.

1991   Shafia Monroe founds the International Center for Traditional Childbearing, an organization focused on the care of pregnant women of color and their families, with a focus on creating more midwives and doulas of color.

1991   The Midwifery Education and Accreditation Council (MEAC), formed by the National Coalition of Midwifery Educators, is officially recognized by the U.S. Department of Education as an accrediting agency for direct-entry midwifery education and institutions.

1992   The North American Registry of Midwives (NARM) is founded and sets the standards for the certified professional midwife (CPM) credential.

1992   Doulas of North America, or DONA International, is founded as the world's first and largest doula-certifying organization. The first president of the organization was Penny Simkin, who in the 1980s formed a partnership with other doulas and medical professionals that eventually led to DONA International. It was the first organization of its kind to train and certify doulas, marking the start of doulas as a professional position. The organization exists to support doulas professionally and to advance the vision of a doula for every person who wants one.

1995   The American Pregnancy Association, formerly known as America's Crisis Pregnancy Helpline, is established by Mike and Anne Sheaffer, who initially set up a hotline to support pregnant people seeking an adoptive couple for their babies. After receiving over 1,000 calls from people facing unplanned pregnancies with nowhere else to turn, the couple recognized this unfulfilled need in society and wanted to set up a confidential crisis line to allow people to receive the help they needed. In 2003, the helpline became the American Pregnancy Association, which became a foundation of health services for anyone in need, including education, research, advocacy, public policy and community awareness as well as a leading organization for reproductive and pregnancy health information.

1996   Citizens for Midwifery is founded as a grassroots non-profit volunteer organization by a group of mothers to promote the Midwives Model of Care, or the best kind of care for pregnancy and childbirth, including safety, respect, cost-effectiveness, and promotion of health- and family-centered care. The goal was to ensure that this model of care would be available to all childbearing women.

1997   SisterSong Women of Color Reproductive Justice Collective is formed by 16 organizations of women of color from four small communities, including Indigenous, Black, Latina, and Asian American. They recognized that women have the right and responsibility to represent themselves and their communities, especially due to the pressing need to advance the perspectives and needs of women of color. SisterSong is a Southern–based national organization that seeks to build an effective network of people and organizations to improve the institutional policies and systems that have a serious impact on marginalized communities and their reproductive lives.

1998   The United States Breastfeeding Committee (USBC) is an independent nonprofit organization that was formed in 1998 in response to the Innocenti Declaration of 1990, of which the U.S. Agency for International Development was a cosponsor. Among other recommendations, the Innocenti Declaration calls on every nation to establish a multisectoral national breastfeeding committee, which comprises representatives from relevant government departments, nongovernmental organizations, and health professional associations to coordinate national breastfeeding initiatives. The USBC is now a coalition of more than 100 organizations that support its mission to drive collaborative efforts for policy and practices that create a landscape of breastfeeding support across the United States.

2001 The National Association of Certified Professional Midwives (NACPM) is founded as the professional organization for certified professional midwives.

2001 National Advocates for Pregnant Women (NAPW) is founded by Lynn M. Paltrow as a nonprofit organization that works to secure the human and civil rights and health and welfare of all people. Its focus is pregnant and parenting women in particular as well as low-income women, women of color, and drug-using women because these groups are more likely to be targeted for state control and punishment.

2006 The Association of Midwifery Educators (AME) is formed at the Midwives Alliance of North America conference in Baltimore, Maryland. A group of midwifery educators and supporters formed the AME due to the need for midwifery educators to network with one another so they can form connections and collaborations.

2008 Ancient Song Doula Services is founded as an international doula certification organization in Brooklyn, New York, with the goal to offer quality doula services to women of color and low-income families who otherwise would not be able to afford doula care. They work to train a workforce of full spectrum doulas to address health inequities within the communities they want to serve.

2008 In January, the film *The Business of Being Born* is released by filmmaker Abby Epstein and talk show host/actress Ricki Lake to explore the perinatal health care system in the United States. With a focus on New York City, the film reveals the impacts of industrialization, capitalism, and the medicalization of pregnancy and birth in the United States.

2008 Thomas Beatie is the first transgender person to give birth. Thomas conceived a child via artificial insemination because his wife, Nancy, was infertile. They used donor sperm and Thomas's own eggs. In July 2008, Thomas gave birth to a healthy baby girl at the St. Charles Medical Centre in Bend, Oregon.

2009 The Seattle Midwifery School merges with Bastyr University to offer the nation's first accredited direct-entry master of science in midwifery and to deliver innovative training for additional childbirth professions.

2009 Elephant Circle is founded as an organization that provides expertise and support to individuals and groups on HOW and WHAT of birth justice which seeks to dismantle systems of oppression for the liberation of all peoples

2010 On March 10, Amnesty International issues a seminal report entitled *Deadly Delivery: The Maternal Health Care Crisis in the USA*. This report showed that while the United States spends more money than any other country on health care, it ranked 41st in terms of maternal death. The study revealed the many barriers people face in accessing high-quality perinatal health care and highlighted it as a basic human rights issue, as these deaths can be prevented with the proper treatment and care.

2011 The Birth Place Lab in the Division of Midwifery at the University of British Columbia is founded. The lab facilitates projects involving multidisciplinary and community-based research as well as knowledge translation regarding access to high-quality maternity health care. These activities were generated by the Home Birth Summits starting in 2011 and continuing through 2014, where national leaders came together to discuss ways to improve perinatal health care services for people choosing to have home births or use birth centers. Professor Saraswathi Vedam is the principal of the Birth Place Lab and supports many teams of multidisciplinary researchers, who collaborate on projects involving health services, patient experience, provider attitudes, and access to physiologic birth across many birth settings.

2012 August is World Breastfeeding Awareness Month, but the last week of the month is especially important for many women across the country: it is Black Breastfeeding Week, a time specifically dedicated to Black women who choose to breastfeed. The week, founded by Anayah Sangodele-Ayoka, Kimberley Seals Allers, and Kiddada Green in 2012, aims to provide support to the many Black women who do breastfeed and to create a community for breastfeeding Black women to show they are not alone.

2012 The National Association of Certified Professional Midwives (NACPM) releases a "Statement of Strategic Intent to Address Racism and Racial Disparities in Maternity Care in the United States." The statement is a commitment to address racism on an individual, board, and organizational level; people of color in organizational leadership, including the board of directors and staff; and a more representative CPM workforce.

2012 The American College of Nurse-Midwives (ACNM) forms a Diversification and Inclusion Task Force to understand its strengths and barriers in this area and to develop strategies to become a more diverse and inclusive organization.

2012 Inspired by the 2011 International Confederation of Midwives (ICM) Global Standards for Midwifery Education, Regulation, and Association (MERA), the U.S. Midwifery Education, Regulation, and Association (US MERA) is formed to strengthen U.S. midwifery.

Representatives of national midwifery associations, credentialing bodies and education accreditation agencies met to establish a new vision and mission to help increase access to high quality with a unified voice for all issues affecting midwifery education, certification, accreditation, and regulation. These organizations included the American College of Nurse-Midwives (ACNM), the Accreditation Commission for Midwifery Education (ACME), the American Midwifery Certification Board (AMCB), the Midwifery Education and Accreditation Council (MEAC), the Midwives Alliance of North America (MANA), the National Association of Certified Professional Midwives (NACPM), and the North American Registry of Midwives (NARM). The founding group included Katherine Camacho Carr, CNM, PhD, FACNM (ACME); Jo

Anne Myers-Ciecko, MPH (MEAC); Cara Krulewitch, CNM, PhD, FACN (AMCB); Brynne Potter, CPM (NARM); Cathy Collins-Fulea, CNM, MSN, FACNM (ACNM); Geradine Simkins, CNM, MSN (MANA); and Mary Lawlor, CPM, LM, MA (NACPM). From US MERA's founding, Shafia Monroe, MPH, fought for the International Center for Traditional Childbearing (ICTC) to representation on the coalition. This was achieved in 2016. The American College of Obstetricians and Gynecologists endorsed the US MERA agreements.

2014   The Birth Rights Bar Association (BRBA) is founded. Pregnant people are frequently denied their right to make informed decisions about the health care they receive during birth and other reproductive health services; this lack of informed consent constitutes a human rights violation that could be attributed to States and national health systems. BRBA provides legal education, networking, and research, and collaborates on institutional legal advocacy efforts.

2016   On April 13, Kira Johnson, a Black woman, died at Cedars-Sinai Medical Center in Los Angeles 10 hours after giving birth to her second son. She was a 39-year-old mother of two who bled to death after a routine scheduled cesarean section. While her symptoms worsened and she was classified as a medical emergency, she did not receive surgery until hours later, where she died immediately after physicians found three-and-a-half liters of blood in her abdomen. Charles Johnson, Kira's husband, started a nonprofit organization called 4Kira-4Moms to generate awareness and prevent more deaths, as he believed that if his wife had been white she would still be alive. According to U.S. statistics on maternal mortality rate, Black women are 209 percent more likely to die than white women. Charles Johnson also filed a lawsuit against the hospital, and he testified before Congress and worked with them to pass HR1318, the Preventing Maternal Deaths Act of 2018, which provides funding to states to have maternal mortality review committees.

2017   The Maternal Health and Accountability Act is sponsored by former Senator Heidi Heitkamp. This bill directs the U.S. Department of Health & Human Services (HHS) to establish programs to make grants to states for the purpose of reviewing pregnancy-related and pregnancy-associated deaths, to establish and sustain a maternal mortality review committee to review relevant information, to ensure the state departments of health plan for ongoing health care provider education to improve maternal care, to disseminate a case abstraction form to aid information collection for review, and to provide the public disclosure of the information included in state reports.

2018   The Black Mamas Matter Alliance is founded by a steering committee that includes Angela Doyinsola Aina, Elizabeth Dawes Gay, Joia Crear-Perry, Kwajelyn Jackson, and Monica Simpson. This was the result of a partnership project between two different organizations, the Center for Reproductive Rights (CRR) and SisterSong Women of Color Reproductive Justice Collective (SisterSong), which began in 2013. Monica Simpson of SisterSong, Katrina Anderson of CRR, and Elizabeth Dawes Gay brought together various experts and activists who shared their concern for Black maternal health. Their partnership was a collaboration of stories collected about the struggles and obstacles faced by Southern Black women when it comes to accessing maternal health care. In 2018, this committee of women was formed to turn the Black Mamas Matter Alliance into its own entity. Their mission is to advocate, drive research, build power, and shift culture for Black maternal health, rights, and justice. Also in 2018, BMMA founded Black Maternal Health Week which takes place every year from April 11–17. The month of April is recognized in the United States as National Minority Health Month—a month-long initiative to advance health equity across the country on behalf of all racial and ethnic minorities.

2018   On April 13, the International Center for Traditional Childbearing officially changes its name to the National

Association to Advance Black Birth (NAABB). The NAABB continues ICTC's 30-year legacy in the promotion of midwives, doulas, and training programs to improve the overall care of Black women, persons, and infants. The name change from ICTC to NAABB signaled a more primary focus on addressing issues with birthing in the Black community throughout the United States.

2018   Although Dr. J. Marion Sims is known to some as the "father of gynecology," he is known to others as a torturer who performed experimental surgeries on enslaved Black women without the use of anesthesia. On April 17, his statue is removed from Central Park. New York City's Public Design Commission unanimously voted to take the statue down. Mayor Bill de Blasio ordered that the statue be removed the next day. This was due to a wave of protests against U.S. statues that commemorate controversial persons. It took eight years of protests, activism, and over 26,000 signatures from the local community to finally remove the 80-year-old statue.

2018   On August 22, the Maternal CARE Act is introduced by Senator Kamala Harris. Also known as Maternal Care Access and Reducing Emergencies, this bill requires the U.S. Department of Health & Human Services (HHS) to award grants to health professional training programs. These programs address implicit bias in the practice of gynecology and obstetrics.

2020   Congresswoman Lauren Underwood, Congresswoman Alma Adams, and members of the Black Maternal Health Caucus first introduce the Black Maternal Health Momnibus Act to fill gaps in existing legislation to comprehensively address every dimension of the Black maternal health crisis in the United States, including support for incarcerated women and women veterans.

2020   Planned Parenthood of Greater New York announces its intent to remove Margaret Sanger's name from their Manhattan Health Center following an organizational commitment to become an anti-racist organization and incorporate principles of race equity into decision-making at every level.

2020   The National Association to Advance Black Birth issues the Black Birthing Bill of Rights, which states, "At NAABB we believe that all Black women and birthing persons are entitled to respectful, equitable, and high-quality pre- and postpartum care. The Black Birthing Bill of Rights is a resource for every black person that engages in maternity care. We want each black woman and birthing person to know their rights and to have the tools to confidently exercise these rights. The Bill of Rights also serves as guidance for government programs, hospitals, maternity providers and others as they transform their policies, procedures, and practices to meet the needs of Black birthing people."

2020   The Black women–led SACRED Birth in the Time of COVID-19 team launches a landmark study with Black mothers and Black birthing people to share information about their patient experiences in hospital settings during labor, birth, and postpartum in six key areas: safety, autonomy, communication, racism, empathy, and dignity.

2020   Actress Crissy Teigen publishes a moving personal narrative about the circumstances surrounding giving birth to her stillborn baby boy and explains the importance of documenting her experience. Her story sparked continued conversation regarding the need to destigmatize pregnancy loss.

2020   The National Birth Equity Collaborative releases *The Birth Equity Agenda: A Blueprint for Reproductive Health and Wellbeing.*

This glossary provides a list of key terms commonly used in the context of discussing pregnancy and birth in the United States. Many are evidence of the medicalization of pregnancy and birth discussed throughout this book.

abortion   The consenting termination of a pregnancy, most commonly in the first 20 weeks of gestation, before the embryo or fetus could survive outside of the womb.

adoption   Generally means to "take as one's own"; in this context, it refers to the legal transfer of parenthood from the biological parents to the adopting parents.

assisted reproductive technologies (ART)   Originally termed "artificial," the word was changed to the more care-oriented language of "assisted"; the technologies include in vitro fertilization (IVF; joining egg and sperm outside of the body), embryo transfer, and egg and sperm freezing, among others.

cervix   The cylinder of fibromuscular tissue at the base of the uterus; in labor, the cervix dilates, or opens, and connects the uterus to the vagina as part of the birth canal.

cesarean section   A surgical procedure by which a viable fetus is removed through incisions made in the abdominal wall and the uterus.

concordant care   Sometimes used to mean shared decision making between providers and patients, the term is increasingly used to mean a shared identity—cultural, racial, ethnic, gender, sexuality, etc.

demedicalization The process in which a condition or behavior becomes defined as a natural, physiologic condition or process rather than a medical condition or illness.

doula A trained care provider who gives continuous physical, emotional, and informational support before, during, and after childbirth. Doulas may provide other care supports for infertility or death and dying.

embryo An embryo is the early stage of human development in which organs and critical body systems are formed. The embryonic period is approximately between the third and eighth week after conception.

epidural An injection in the lower back into the area just outside of the membrane that protects the spinal cord, which causes numbness, an inability to feel, in the lower half of the body.

episiotomy A surgical incision in the perineum, the skin between the vagina and the rectum, to widen the birth outlet. It has been repeatedly proven to create more tearing, pain, and other iatrogenic damage than the potential tear it was intended to avoid.

fetus The embryo is considered a fetus usually from the ninth week after conception, until the time of birth. During this period, the baby's organs and critical body systems continue to develop.

iatrogenic Illness or disease caused by medical management.

induction of labor When labor does not begin spontaneously, it may be induced via medical or mechanical means. This has become considerably more common in recent years, contributing to the rise of longer and more painful labors and the ultimate rise in cesarean sections.

infertility Generally defined as not conceiving after a year or more of regular unprotected sex.

lactation   The secretion of milk from the mammary glands; more commonly known as *breastfeeding* or *chestfeeding*.

lactation consultant   A trained care provider who provides support, information, and help for parents who are breastfeeding.

medicalization   The process in which a condition or behavior becomes defined as a medical condition requiring a medical intervention or in which the definition of an illness is broadened to cover a wider population.

midwife   The word *midwife* has its root in Old English for "with" (mid) "woman" (wife); the midwife was the woman in the community who was responsible for helping in childbirth. In many languages, this is called the "wise woman" (e.g., French, *sage femme*; Dutch, *vroedvrouw*). All midwives practice using the Midwives Model of Care:

- Monitoring the physical, psychological, and social well-being of the mother throughout the childbearing cycle.
- Providing the mother with individualized education, counseling, and prenatal care, continuous hands-on assistance during labor and delivery, and postpartum support.
- Minimizing technological interventions.
- Identifying and referring women who require obstetrical attention.

The application of this woman-centered model of care has been proven to reduce the incidence of birth injury, trauma, and cesarean section.

Copyright © 1996–2008, Midwifery Task Force, Inc., All Rights Reserved.

miscarriage   The spontaneous, nonplanned, an unintended end of a pregnancy before viability,; in medical terms, this is sometimes called *spontaneous abortion*.

neonate   A baby in the first 28 days after birth.

NICU   The Neonatal Intensive Care Unit is a hospital ward dedicated to the care of seriously ill or premature neonates.

nosocomial   A disease, usually an infection, that develops in a hospital and infects patients. The original understanding came from the work of Semmelweis, who saw that puerperal fever, or postpartum infection, occurred among people treated in hospitals by physicians; handwashing was introduced to reduce occurrence.

Ob-Gyn   Obstetrics and gynecology is the surgical specialty within medicine devoted to the care of pregnancy and birth and the diagnosis and treatment of diseases of the female reproductive system as well as other issues defined as women's health issues, including menopause, conception, and contraception.

pediatrics   The medical specialty devoted to the care of infants and children through adolescence. Neonatology is the subspecialty for newborn care and illness.

perinatal health worker   A trained care provider who works with people in pregnancy and postpartum to provide direct perinatal care and support, including nutrition, lactation, and breastfeeding support.

placenta   The organ that develops in pregnancy, implanting within the wall of the uterus and connecting, via the umbilical cord, the pregnant person and the embryo/fetus, supplying nutrients and removing waste. It is known as the *afterbirth* expelled following the birth of the baby.

premature birth   A birth before the 37th week of gestation. The baby is referred to as a *premature baby* or *preemie*. The earlier the birth, the more intensive the care may be needed.

Reproductive Justice   A theoretical framework and care practice that links reproductive rights with social justice. It is the human right to maintain personal bodily autonomy, have children, not have children, and parent one's children in safe and sustainable communities.

stillbirth   The death of a fetus or baby after *viability*, which may occur before, during, or at the time of birth.

surrogacy An arrangement, often supported by a legal agreement, whereby a person consents to birth a child for another person or persons, who will become the child's parent(s) after birth.

viability Generally means the ability to live; in pregnancy, it refers to the point at which the fetus could survive outside of the womb, usually understood to be after 20 weeks of gestation.

zygote The single cell formed when the sperm and ovum join; as these cells replicate, it becomes a blastocyst, and then it differentiates further and becomes a developing embryo at approximately two to three weeks after conception.

Note: Page numbers followed by *t* indicate tables and *f* indicate figures.

About the Authors

Keisha L. Goode, PhD, lectures in sociology and criminology at the State University of New York College at Old Westbury and in sociology and women's and gender studies at the City University of New York, Lehman College. Her work is centered on issues related to pregnancy and childbirth in the United States, with specific attention to Black midwifery. She is the first public member of the board of directors of the National Association of Certified Professional Midwives and is currently serving as the board vice president.

Barbara Katz Rothman, PhD, is a professor of sociology, women's studies, and public health at the City University of New York, Baruch College and Graduate Center. She has been working on issues related to pregnancy and birth throughout her career. Her books include *A Bun in the Oven: How the Food and Birth Movements Resist Industrialization*, *In Labor*, *The Tentative Pregnancy*, *Recreating Motherhood*, *The Book of Life*, *Weaving a Family: Untangling Race and Adoption*, and *Laboring On*. She recently held the Fulbright-Saastamoinen Distinguished Chair in Health Sciences at the University of Eastern Finland and was past president of Sociologists for Women in Society as well as the Society for the Study of Social Problems and the Eastern Sociological Society. She is most proud to be the recipient of the Midwifing the Movement Award from the Midwives Alliance of North America.